Women Theorists of Psychotherapy and Counseling

Women Theorists of Psychotherapy and Counseling

Lynn Bohecker, Kirsten LaMantia
and Holly H. Wagner

LEXINGTON BOOKS
Lanham • Boulder • New York • London

Published by Lexington Books
An imprint of The Rowman & Littlefield Publishing Group, Inc.
4501 Forbes Boulevard, Suite 200, Lanham, Maryland 20706
www.rowman.com

6 Tinworth Street, London SE11 5AL, United Kingdom

British Library Cataloguing in Publication Information Available

Library of Congress Cataloging-in-Publication Data

Library of Congress Control Number: 2020950409

ISBN: 978-1-7936-0847-5 (cloth)
ISBN: 978-1-7936-0848-2 (electronic)

Contents

Introduction

The Necessity and Subsequent Invisibility of Women Theorists

Crack open any theories of counseling and psychotherapy textbook, find the table of contents, and you will find a long list of men. Men have long been considered both the ideal authors and the subjects of theories. Theories are written by men, for men, with little attention to how the theories reflect the everyday lived experiences of women and other marginalized populations. However, research suggests that a Eurocentric, masculine approach is not, in fact, the most efficacious framework when working with minority, marginalized, or oppressed populations (Sue & Sue, 2013). It would be far-fetched to believe that women theorists have not existed. It is far more likely that the theories and contributions of women to the fields of counseling and psychotherapy have been diminished and downplayed. If we take a historical view and apply a social constructionist understanding of knowledge to the field, we see that women contributors, theorists, have been silenced and sidelined, and their work has been stolen for the benefit of their male counterparts. Throughout this book you will learn about women who have significantly contributed to counseling and psychotherapy. Their backgrounds, contexts, and stories will facilitate an understanding of their unique perspectives. Their significant contributions will be highlighted and cited to show how their voices, ideas, and new ways of thinking have shaped our current ideas of mental health and wellness. Though these women theorists are minimally or not discussed in other books, in our book they are the focus of attention. We amplify their voices and demonstrate how their work has influenced and changed the course of counseling and psychotherapy.

WHY IS THIS BOOK NEEDED?

Counseling and psychotherapy practices are shaped by theory in an interactive relationship. British and North American middle-class values, ideas, concepts, and social standards have long permeated academia impacting knowledge in the social sciences (Joseph et al., 1990; Katz, 1985). Identified as Eurocentrism, this bias colonized alternative sources of knowledge offered by women and non-Europeans. Eurocentric bias is present in psychological assumptions, impacting training and application to the mental health of other racial groups and women (Joseph et al., 1990; Miller, 2012; Sue & Sue, 2013). Counseling and psychological theories and practice have been criticized by minority and feminist scholars as culturally encapsulated, lacking in multicultural relevance, and conceptualized in Eurocentric individualistic terms (Sue & Sue, 2013).

Jereb (1982) suggested that counseling theories were inadequate for both working with and subsequently helping Black clients. The same was said for Asian Americans, Latinx people, and lesbian, gay, bisexual, and transgender (LGBT) communities (Crethar et al., 2008; Erford, 2014; Hays, 2008; Sue & Sue, 2013). Similarly, what may be effective for men does not automatically apply to women (Miller, 2012). Counselors may acknowledge the influences of differences between themselves and clients related to gender and culture, however "many counselors continue to be unaware of the fact that the profession has at its core an inherent set of cultural values and norms by which clients are judged" (Katz, 1985, p. 615). Eurocentric male cultural values provide the foundation of norms for counseling and psychology professions.

Theories about human behavior are the result of individuals observing other people. When viewing others, the position of the viewer is through a unique perspective grounded in experiences, values, beliefs, and the societal and political norms in which they live. Theorists interpret their observations of others, and their context and perspective influence those interpretations. It would be highly unlikely that Eurocentric males would be able to capture effectively or interpret accurately the behaviors of all people, particularly women and populations of non-European origins.

Eurocentrism benefits the dominant group, White males, and there is little incentive to share those benefits with women and people of color. The benefits for White men have been highlighted by McIntosh (1988) and labeled "White privilege." Bulhan (1985) explained that the impact of the privilege for this dominant group is that the experiences and opinions of White males are the only or most valid experiences in the world. The result, therefore, is that the opinions and perspectives of women are not considered as important, manifesting in the systemic silencing of women. Historically, women have been discouraged from working apart from managing a home and raising children.

Women who were able to pursue higher education and career employment were and still are often paid less than their male counterparts. It is well documented that women's talents and accomplishments are minimized, often go unnoticed, or even worse, taken by a man and promoted as his own.

Women have been sidelined in psychological theory development through the traditional western roles of wife and mother. Women who ventured into counseling and psychotherapy theory development were minimized and viewed as crossing rigid male-female role boundaries and, therefore, not seen as credible or taken seriously. The result of Eurocentrism in relation to the creation and development of theories in counseling and psychotherapy was a preference for the White men and the subordination of women and people of color (Miller, 2012). Therefore, there is a compelling need to hear from women. Ultimately, a more expansive perspective is needed when describing those who have contributed their theoretical lenses to our current body of counseling knowledge.

This book focuses on explaining some of the theories of psychotherapy and counseling created by women. In reading this book, your understanding of some cultures and therapeutic approaches will be broadened. In addition to understanding each of the theories, you will begin to understand the political and social climate during which each theory was created. Some of the women highlighted in this book did not have access to the resources or public outlets needed to make their work known. Others had to contend with their famous fathers' and/or husbands' influences too. This book will enhance your ability to recognize how social and historical contexts not only impact the work done at a particular time but also how individuals from marginalized communities can create, expand upon, and dismantle counseling and psychotherapy theories during times of duress.

STRUCTURE OF EACH CHAPTER

Before you continue reading this book, it may be helpful for you to understand the layout of the following chapters. Each chapter in this book discusses women and their theories of wellness, treatment, and ways of being. Each chapter is authored by one of the three editors of this book, so you may find that the tone and voice of the writing vary. Additionally, we experienced a range of available information from large volumes of work to a minimal amount. As the editors, we believe a variation in each chapter is one simultaneously an indication of how work produced by women can be lost and an opportunity for each chapter author to integrate her unique voice and writing style. Just as theories of counseling and psychotherapy must not rely on a monolithic narrative, so too is it necessary to avoid bringing only one voice to the proverbial pedagogical table. Hearing from individuals who inhabit various cultural identities can help you begin to better understand your own views, especially those pertaining to how humans interact with the world, how the world interacts with them, and the countless ways that humans experience the journey to wellness.

While each of the chapters is unique in some facets, the chapters have a consistent skeleton. The major subsections of each chapter are Theorist Biography, Key Concepts and Utilization of Theory, and Subversive Nature of Theory. The following are short introductions to the various subsections.

Theorist Biography

You will find a brief biography of a theorist at the beginning of each chapter. Special attention is given to childhood, family dynamics and the sociopolitical climate surrounding the theorist and the creation of her theory. This subsection gives you context for understanding her theory by introducing you to its founder and her evolution as a person before you uncover her theoretical vision in the subsequent subsection.

Key Concepts and Utilization of Theory

This subsection introduces the main ideas of the theory and gives you a sense of its distinguishing aspects. What is the essence of this theory? What makes it unique? Why was it created? These questions are addressed as you begin reading about the theoretical lens. Then the key concepts of any theory must be explored in order to ascertain what makes a theory unique and viewed as important or special and be considered accordingly. This subsection deconstructs the theory's main terminology and gives you a clear understanding of the key conceptual pieces that comprise the theory as a whole. The therapeutic process works differently depending on the theoretical underpinnings or lens of the practitioner. This subsection elucidates the process of change according to the theory under discussion and thereby demonstrates how the introductory knowledge and key concepts that were previously presented are applied.

Subversive Nature of Theory

This subsection explores the context and how the theory impacted the helping profession during times in history that were dominated by men. What did it mean to have a theory presented by a woman? How did a woman's voice affect how the theory was received? What impact did this theory have on the helping profession as a whole?

IMPACT OF THIS BOOK

Now you know why we wrote this book, why the work of women theorists needs to be recovered, and how the book is laid out. But what do we hope will happen as you read this book? We hope that you will gain a broader understanding of how women have contributed to the fields of counseling, psychotherapy, and mental health. Beyond advancing the work of well-known male theorists, women have created their own theories that have shaped the mental health work of the twenty-first century. In order for you to become more multiculturally competent, it is imperative that you understand the worldviews of other cultures. If you only study the work of White men, you will only know the ways in which White men both view the world and view mental wellness. By learning from women, entirely new worldviews will be opened to you.

REFERENCES

Crethar, H. C., Rivera, E. T., & Nash, S. (2008). In search of common threads: Linking multicultural, feminist, and social justice counseling paradigms. *Journal of Counseling & Development*, *86*(3), 269–278. doi:10.1002/j.1556-6678.2008.tb00509.x

Erford, B. T. (2014). *Orientation to the Counseling Profession: Advocacy, Ethics, and Essential Professional Foundations* (2nd edition). Pearson.

Hays, P. A. (2008). *Addressing Cultural Complexities in Practice: Assessment, Diagnosis, and Therapy* (2nd edition). American Psychological Association.

Jereb, R. J. (1982). Assessing the adequacy of counseling theories for use with Black clients. *Counseling and Values*, *27*(1), 17–26. doi:10.1002/j.2161-007X.1982.tb01121.x

Joseph, G. G., Reddy, V., & Searle-Chatterjee, M. (1990). Eurocentrism in the social sciences. *Race & Class, 31*(4), 1–26. doi:10.1177/030639689003100401

Katz, J. H. (1985). The sociopolitical nature of counseling. *The Counseling Psychologist, 13*(4), 615–624. doi:10.1177%2F0011000085134005

Miller, J. B. (2012). *Toward a New Psychology of Women.* Beacon Press.

Sue, D. W., & Sue, D. (2013). *Counseling the Culturally Diverse: Theory and Practice* (6th edition). John Wiley & Sons.

Chapter 1

Developmental Theorists

One of the most interesting aspects of studying the women involved in improving our understanding of developmental psychology is the women's diverging views on the nature of the self as it pertains to both the public and the private spheres. Despite operating in cultures that offered women only limited access to advanced educational opportunities, each of the women presented in this chapter not only pursued higher education in some form but also went on to make significant impacts in her professional field of study: developmental psychology. Even more striking is that each of the women came to very different conclusions regarding the challenges and benefits of feminism. Building on each other's work, the women theorists in this chapter described the importance of psychologically healthy women, and specifically mothers, during the developmental process. Margaret Mahler (1897–1985) was the first to include the mother when treating severely disturbed children, Mary Ainsworth (1913–1999), was instrumental in providing the research to support attachment theory, and Carol Gilligan (1936–) inspired the passage of the 1993 Gender Equity in Education Act. Talk therapy and the direct effects of anti-Semitism are essential threads in the developmental theories each woman eventually created.

THEORIST BIOGRAPHY: MARGARET MAHLER

Margaret Mahler (née Schönberger) was born to Jewish parents on May 10, 1897, in Sopron, West Hungary, fewer than forty miles from Vienna, Austria. Anti-Jewish sentiment in the region made an early impact on Mahler as her grandmother came to live with the family due to the threat of a pogrom in

Esterhazy, Hungary (Stepansky, 1988). By the summer of 1914, these tensions would become a contributing factor in the eruption of World War I.

Mahler felt a sense of pride in her father's choice to send her to a private primary school to ensure she received the best educational foundation available. Anti-Semitism was not recognized as a serious threat in Austro-Hungarian spaces, including the army, at that time. Censorship was used extensively during the initial years of World War I in Austria because the Austrian government wanted to maintain Jewish support in defeating Russia. In these areas, people of Jewish descent held significant roles. These people included Ferenc Heltai (1861–1913), who was the mayor of Budapest when war was declared. Meanwhile, converted Jew Samuel von Hazai (1851–1942) headed the Hungarian war ministry (Bihari, 2016).

Her father's encouragement of Mahler's academic interests stood in sharp contrast to what Mahler experienced as a lack of support or even interest from her mother, with whom she had a difficult relationship (Stepansky, 1988). Mahler strongly felt that her mother favored her younger sibling. She would later identify this as key in the development of her anger toward her mother and deep resentment toward her sister. Support from her father in being for herself "all the man she would ever need" formed the basis of a bond that Mahler would later identify as the primary challenge she faced in the development of her identity as a woman and a professional (Stepansky, 1988). However, there were challenges Mahler had to contend with as the only female child of Jewish descent in her private elementary school. The difficulties surfaced within her first weeks at the school when a pamphlet was sent to each of her peers advising students not to talk to her because the Israelites crucified Jesus Christ, in response to her presence.

With her father's continued encouragement, Mahler moved to Budapest, living with her maternal aunt while completing her two years at the High School for Daughters (Mahler, 1977). Such levels of educational achievement were rare for women; indeed, Mahler was only the second girl to have left her home district to seek a high school education. The local school was highly respected; however, it did not accept women. During high school Mahler met several influential men, including Hungarian psychoanalyst Sándor Ferenczi. His influence led Mahler to read Sigmund Freud's *Three Essays on Sexuality* (1962) at the age of nineteen. Mahler subsequently became intrigued by psychology and Freud's concept of the unconscious.

After completing her education at the High School for Daughters, Mahler enrolled at the University of Budapest in fall 1916. There she began art history studies, which she thought an appropriately feminine course of study. However, her earlier interest in medicine, coupled with highly conflicted feelings about her father's encouragement to focus on academics rather than her relationships with peers and potential suitors, led her in January 1917 to switch to medical studies (Mahler, 1977). Her first three semesters of medical school at the University of Munich went well academically. However, the rising economic and anti-Semitic tensions that would eventually lead to the collapse of the Weimar Republic, a parliamentary democracy established in the defeated Germany after World War I, prompted her to transfer to the University of Jena in spring 1920. The last years of the Weimar Republic were plagued by political deadlock, increasing political street violence, increasing anti-Semitic attacks and accusations of Jewish men undermining the military in Hungary but that Mahler fought her circumstances to nonetheless graduate cum laude in 1922.

After graduation, Mahler began working as a physician. Her interest in psychology grew, leading her to pursue training in child psychiatry and psychoanalytic techniques. Training at the Vienna Psychoanalytic Institute proved to be a difficult process for Mahler, as evidenced by her training analysis. At the beginning of her training analysis in 1926, Mahler worked with Helene Deutsch; she then switched to August Aichorn (who became her lover; Mahler, 1979). She ultimately completed the training analysis with Willi Hoffer, becoming a certified analyst in 1933. This was also the year of the death of her good friend and longtime advisor Ferenczi. In a union she described as "a pseudosolution to psychological problems that were still not fully resolved" (Mahler, 1979, p. 79), Mahler married her husband Paul in 1936. Mahler and her husband escaped to Britain and then the United States with the help of the international psychoanalytic community.

By 1939 the couple had settled into New York despite some resistance from the then-current members of the New York Psychoanalytic Society. In the end, Mahler joined the Institute of Human Development, the Educational Institute, and the New York Psychoanalytic Society with Benjamin Spock. The Institute supported her continued work, which focused increasingly on clinical studies of childhood psychosis. She felt that her earlier research with Clemons von Pirquet's clinic showed how devastating a sterile, detached caregiver connection during early child development could be to very ill infants. However, she also observed how Moll's institute could produce a "therapeutically potent" effect on this same population through its emphasis on emotional connection and engagement (Stepansky, 1988, p. 82).

Mahler's father died one month before the German invasion of Hungary in 1944. During the period of illness that preceded Mahler's father's death, the *Bürgermeister* (mayor) of Sopron suggested that Mahler's mother leave immediately with Mahler's husband and his nurse. She declined the suggestion repeatedly, believing that they would all do well in Sopron where the family was firmly established and well respected. Eugenie Wiener Schönberger died in Auschwitz one year later, in summer 1944. Stepansky (1988) wrote,

> In point of fact, the entire Jewish community of Sopron, Dr. [Margaret] Mahler's native village, was virtually wiped out by the Nazis. At the time of the German occupation of March 1944, the town had 1,856 Jewish residents. Over the course of the next two months, 1,470 of these Jews were deported to concentration camps, 40 were arrested, 286 were conscripted for forced labor, 55 were infirm elderly, and 5 were declared "honorary citizens" and allowed to remain. (p. 156)

In 1950 Manuel Furer joined Mahler in founding the Masters Children's Center in Manhattan as part of Mount Sinai Hospital. It was there that Mahler developed the tripartite treatment model (Mahler & Furer, 1960). This approach was among the first to include the mother in the treatment of the child. In her work with deeply disturbed children, Mahler observed that the child's environment is an important factor. Based on this, she began to study the connections between mothers and their children through observations of children's reactions to brief separations from their mothers. These first structured investigations of separation allowed Mahler to recognize that separation-individuation could be understood as the beginning of an infant's psychological life. Her work clarified the concept of a developmental process through which infants gradually develop self-awareness and self-reflection, ultimately facilitating increasing levels of autonomy and individuality. In recognition of Mahler's work, Barnard College awarded Mahler the Barnard Medal of Distinction, the highest award given by the college, in 1980. Mahler died on October 2, 1985, at eighty-eight years of age.

Key Concepts and Utilization of Theory

Through her research with disturbed children (Mahler et al., 1973), Mahler clarified the importance of the connection to a primary caregiver in an infant's development of an autonomous sense of self. She came to understand the development of an autonomous self as an intrapsychic separation-individuation process composed of successive stages, each indicating the child's internal "separation" from the caregiver. Infants increasingly come to understand themselves as separate from their primary caregivers, ultimately developing an ability to recognize themselves as distinct individuals with distinct points of view and senses of self (Bergman, 1999). Looking at the child's behavior during observable temporary separation experiences as a behavioral manifestation of internal psychological progress, or a lack of progress, is an original and significant contribution Mahler made to attachment theory, and in particular, to its conceptualization of mother-child relationships.

John Bowlby, a founder of attachment theory, viewed a toddler's attachment behaviors (Coates, 2004) as a product of instinctive reactivity. He, along with most early attachment theorists, believed that all young children exhibit these behaviors in some way based on the need to gain nourishment from their caregivers. Thus, the behaviors are not species-specific but are instead indicative of a survival need. Earlier research experiences with Bowlby as well as Mahler's own private practice as a child psychiatrist led Mahler to disagree. Mahler understood separation-individuation to be an internal or intrapsychic process that could not be directly observed but could be inferred (Mahler et al., 1973, p. 23). Adopting a decidedly Freudian theoretical perspective, she described the pre-separation-individuation state of symbiosis as a distinctly human condition. Out of this uniquely human state, separation and individuation are achieved as a way of managing tension by bringing the infant back to a state of psychological equilibrium prior to the emergence of the child's ego, which eventually allows the child to initiate self-comfort (Mahler et al., 1973). In *The Psychological Birth of the Human Infant* (Mahler et al., 1973), Mahler described the phases initially identified through this research:

1. Normal autistic phase: The first few weeks during which the infant appears oblivious to the outside world. Most of their time is spent sleeping.
2. Normal symbiotic phase: This phase lasts until the child is about five months old and visually recognizes their mother. The child still sees themselves as indistinguishable from the mother.
3. Separation-individuation phase: The infant begins to interact with individuals in their environment. This phase is divided into the following sub-phases:
   a. Hatching (from five to ten months): The infant uses the primary caregiver for orientation as the infant begins to move away from the caregiver and to interact more with the environment.
   b. Practicing (from ten to sixteen months): The child begins moving independently (crawling and then walking) to investigate the environment independent of the caregiver.
   c. Reproachment (from sixteen to twenty-four months): The toddler experiences increased anxiety related to distance from the primary caregiver and so attempts to re-establish the connection and return to the former sense of emotional equilibrium. As the child gains language skills, additional ego resources begin to develop, leading the child back toward external environmental exploration.

Subversive Nature of Theory

While women including Sigmund Freud's daughter Anna Freud and peers such as Melanie Klein were engaged with Freud's talk therapy from its beginnings, women were generally not seen as leaders in the professional sphere. Mahler's work challenged the basis of Jean Piaget's theory of object permanence as well as Bowlby's understanding of attachment theory, both of which involved recognizing the behavior of human children as based solely on non-species-specific survival needs. As a result, she was able to explore the developmental challenge the infant faces when the primary caregiver is not visually present to the infant. It became clear to Mahler that when out of sight, the caregiver ceases to exist for the pre-separation-individuation phase infant. As the child matures, their visual capacities increase, allowing their perception of their primary caregiver to become increasingly clear. This allows the infant to observe and then internalize a visual image of the caregiver. Mahler's research suggests that a child who develops a positive internalized image of an independent, yet empathetic caregiver is likely to use that foundation as a basis for a positive sense of self when transitioning to adulthood.

THEORIST BIOGRAPHY: MARY AINSWORTH

Mary Ainsworth was born Mary Salter on December 1, 1913, in Glendale, Ohio. Both of her parents were originally from Pennsylvania. Her parents met at Dickinson College and graduated from there (Ainsworth, 1983). Her father earned a master's degree in history, and her mother settled into homemaking for the family, which eventually grew into childcare for Ainsworth and her two younger sisters. In 1918, the family moved to Toronto, Canada, due to her father's company transfer. Ainsworth showed academic promise early in her elementary school years, which led her mother to seek supportive materials appropriate to the aspirations Ainsworth's parents held for Ainsworth's future. Ainsworth's parents' expectations of academic excellence (Ainsworth, 1983) matched Ainsworth's pleasure in demonstrating prowess in this area. She would later remark that she thoroughly enjoyed learning, which posed no problems until high school when she pretended to be indifferent to learning in order to ingratiate herself with her peers.

This passion for academic achievement led Ainsworth to develop an affinity for psychology. At fifteen years old, she read William McDougall's *Character and the Conduct of Life* (1927) and became fascinated by the idea that an individual could use self-reflection to better understand feelings and behaviors that once seemed wholly controlled by factors from the external world. This revelation (Ainsworth, 1983) led to Ainsworth's first professional aspiration: to become a psychologist. Years later she reflected on a belief commonly held during that time that suggested psychology held the potential for significant improvement in the quality of life for the vast majority of people. This perspective remained with Ainsworth throughout her life, even during the challenges of the Great Depression.

Ainsworth entered the University of Toronto as an underaged freshman in fall 1929, completing her bachelor's degree in 1935. Given her age, the university mandated what it called a first-year Pass Course. Thus, she could not take psychology courses until the second year. Eventually she was accepted into the honors programs, which provided her with intellectual rigor. It was here that she was introduced to the ideas of William E. Blatz. Blatz (1940) had developed security theory, which suggests that in infancy and early childhood individuals strive to develop a sense of secure dependence on their parents. This is necessary to establish the emotionally stable base from which an individual can develop the courage needed to explore a new and unfamiliar world, replete with both joys and disappointments, and develop effective strategies for coping with that world.

After completing a master's degree in 1936 and a doctorate in 1939, Ainsworth taught at the University of Toronto for several years before Great Britain (and by extension Canada) declared war on Germany in September 1939. Ainsworth refrained from joining the war effort for three years despite watching many of her professors and peers leave the university (Ainsworth, 1983) to move into war-related positions. During this time, she further developed her skills in research design and the utilization of testing instruments for children. After initially immersing herself in teaching and research, she opted to join the Canadian Women's Army Corps in July 1942.

After the end of the war, Ainsworth went back to teaching while volunteering with the Department of Veteran's Affairs hospital, beginning her career as a clinical psychologist. During this period, she accepted a position working with John Bowlby at the Tavistock Research unit. Her work there with maternal separation established the foundation of her future approach to research and theory. In 1950, she married her husband Leonard, a former undergraduate on her research team, moving with him to London where he pursued his doctorate. For two years the couple lived in Uganda, where Ainsworth conducted longitudinal studies that she later published as *Infancy in Uganda: Infant Care and the Growth of Love* (1967). The couple divorced in 1960. Personal concern about the effects of the divorce on her life and work prompted Ainsworth to seek therapy, which spurred her interest in psychoanalytic work. In time she moved on to teach at the University of Virginia from 1975 until her death in 1999 in Charlottesville, Virginia.

Key Concepts and Utilization of Theory

Ainsworth's primary contributions to this new way of looking at child development include a recognition of the need for a child to identify with an attachment figure to support the formation of a secure foundation. This type of foundation is needed as it allows the child to feel safe in exploring their environment. Given the importance of the attachment figure, Ainsworth (Bretherton, 1992) explored the types of interactions that support or inhibit this type of connection. It became increasingly clear to her that the mother's sensitivity and ability to respond to messages from the child, or "maternal sensitivity," greatly impacted attachment patterns between the infant and the mother. In documenting and analyzing structured observations and interviews, Ainsworth provided a wealth of information related to early attachment theory.

Before embarking on her later work on attachment theory, Ainsworth (Bowlby et al., 1956) identified three key relationship patterns among school-aged children returning to their families after extended hospital stays. These included children with strong positive feelings toward their mothers, children with observably ambivalent relationships with their mothers, and children with non-relating or hostile relationships with their mothers.

Ainsworth was impressed by Bowlby's understanding of the behavior of children as motivated by biological structure and physiological needs. Interested in undertaking a research-based examination of this motivation in children, she initiated the first formal, structured study of attachment between infants and mothers. It is important to note that her work predates Bowlby's later publications. Building on concepts from ethology and developmental psychology, Bowlby presented his work to the British Psychoanalytic Society in London in three papers that are now considered foundational: "The Nature of the Child's Tie to His Mother" (1958), "Separation Anxiety" (1959), and "Grief and Mourning in Infancy and Early Childhood" (1960). They are considered the first formal statements in which attachment theory is articulated.

Strange situation. To better elucidate the effects of various forms of attachment on individual behavior, Ainsworth explored reactions to stressful situations through structured observations of children and mothers. In what Ainsworth termed the "strange situation" procedure (Ainsworth & Bell, 1970), researchers observed twenty-six children ranging from twelve to eighteen months old. Each infant and caregiver experienced a series of eight episodes, each lasting for three minutes. In the first episode, the pair enter a laboratory with many toys. After one minute, an unknown person joins them in the laboratory and begins to interact with them. The caregiver leaves the infant with the unknown person for three minutes before returning and comforting the child. The caregiver then leaves a second time, this time leaving the child alone for three minutes. In this second episode, it is the "unknown" person who now enters and attempts to comfort the infant, with the caregiver eventually returning to pick up the child. Based on work in the original Baltimore study (Ainsworth & Wittig, 1969), the infants were identified as fitting into one of three categories: secure, ambivalent-insecure, and avoidant insecure. Each group of infants demonstrated a specific type of attachment relationship with their primary caregivers. Each category represented unique strategies (Ainsworth et al., 1978) in communicating, regulating emotion, and perceiving and responding to stressors.

Anxious-avoidant insecure attachment. Children with the anxious-avoidant insecure attachment style often avoid contact with their caregivers. They tend not to respond to the presence or absence of a caregiver or to explore their surroundings in others' presence. Ainsworth and Bell (1970) suspected that this lack of curiosity masked significant distress.

Secure attachment. Securely attached children explore their surroundings extensively while frequently returning to their caregivers as a safe base. These children interact with strangers in the presence of their caregivers. They tend to become upset when their caregivers leave and are happy to see them return.

Anxious-resistant insecure attachment. Anxious-ambivalent/resistant children appear distressed prior to separation. They often cling to their caregivers upon their departure and find it difficult to return to a sense of emotional equilibrium once their caregivers have returned.

Disorganized/disoriented attachment. Ainsworth eventually agreed with her colleague Mary Main (Main & Solomon, 1986) that a fourth classification was needed to describe infants who seem to have no consistent coping mechanisms in the face of stressors. These children demonstrate a clear desire to be close to their caregivers, yet they then engage in equally strong avoidant behaviors. At times they appear surprised or confused at the return of their primary caregivers.

Subversive Nature of Theory

Ainsworth's extensive experience in research methodology enabled her to conduct the empirical examination needed to evaluate Bowlby's concepts of the processes involved in development from infancy into maturity. She went on to challenge and move beyond his work, clarifying, expanding, and refining attachment theory beyond its early limitations.

Perhaps one of the most subversive aspects of Ainsworth's work in terms of feminist thinking is that she developed a theory emphasizing the importance of maternal empathy and responsiveness. This seems like a particular point of contention with second-wave feminism and its encouragement of women's work outside of the home. Feminist literature noticed the cultural contexts in which Ainsworth developer her theory, namely Eurocentrism and prioritizing men's perspectives, thereby questioning validity. There is also a feminist concern with Ainsworth's work for over emphasizing the mother and that, therefore, there is a disproportionate blame on mothers for children's emotional problems. Feminist scholars questioned the emphasis on early life and the validity of attachment measures (Cox, 2006).

Ainsworth's relationship with her father led her to live a life essentially based on that understanding. She approached child-caregiver interactions with an analytical perspective that enabled her to identify fundamental aspects of this relationship. While some question her focus on the mother, her work highlights the importance of the mother's psychological well-being and its effects on her ability to be sensitive and responsive to the child's needs as a crucial factor in enabling the child to form effective connections to the mother and eventually the larger social environment. Ainsworth said,

> I have sometimes been accused of being out of touch with current changes in life-styles, but I believe that the problem is that infants are perhaps a million or so years out of touch with them. . . . Now, however, the human species has been too successful in that the world is overpopulated; at least some women have been relieved of their age-old responsibilities for at least some period of their lives. There seems little reason to doubt that the intelligence and dedication that women have devoted to their traditional role can now, when not required by that role, be channeled elsewhere without undue hindrance. (Ainsworth, 1983, p. 219)

THEORIST BIOGRAPHY: CAROL GILLIGAN

Carol Gilligan (née Friedman) was born on November 28, 1936, in New York City, New York. As the only child of Jewish lawyer William Friedman and nursery schoolteacher Mabel Caminez, she enjoyed access to a private school education on Manhattan's Upper West Side. In this setting, Gilligan pursued a wide variety of interests (Medea, 2009), including creative arts such as piano and dance. Gilligan went on to graduate summa cum laude with her bachelor's degree in literature from Swarthmore College in 1958. Advanced work at Radcliffe University followed, culminating in a master's degree in clinical psychology in 1960. Gilligan went on to obtain her doctorate in social psychology from Harvard University in 1964. Not long after graduation, she married her husband James, the director of Harvard Medical School's Center for the Study of Violence. Eventually, the couple went on to raise three children: Jonathan Mark, Timothy David, and Christopher James.

Key Concepts and Utilization of Theory

Gilligan began a teaching career at Harvard in 1967. In addition to teaching, she began working with Erik Erikson, a psychologist known for his work on developmental stages and their expression in several cultures. By 1970, Gilligan had landed a spot as a research assistant for Lawrence Kohlberg. While Kohlberg eventually became known for his research on moral development in boys and his theory on the stages of moral development, justice, and rights, Gilligan (Woods, 1996) found her research moving toward moral development in girls. This tendency sprang from interviews Gilligan did with young people concerned about the Vietnam War in general and young women who were contemplating abortions in particular.

The initial disagreement between Kohlberg's notion of morality for all, which was based primarily on his research with boys and a masculine point of view, and Gilligan's growing insistence that his approach failed to capture the realities of women's perspectives brought to light core challenges in scholars' understanding of moral development. This disagreement shaped the development of the field, sparking debate about whether each gender operates from differing understandings of the definition of morality itself. Gilligan pointed out that this difference would lead to disparities in scores on instruments measuring moral development, as noted by Kohlberg. Rather than seeing the scores as indications of moral inferiority, Gilligan (1982) argued that women value and thus focus on relationship needs. Meanwhile, men may focus on justice. Gilligan discussed these differences and the importance of expanding scholars' understanding of how morality is understood, taught, and applied in relation to the social contexts and demands on women.

Ethics of Care

Gilligan's assertion of a female-centered value system with its own definition of morality represented a challenge to existing developmental theories concerning morality. Her ethics of care concept suggests that girls understand themselves through relationships and interactions with others. Thus, they tend to value moral approaches that fall in line with a relational or care-based set of values over the logic-based approaches valued in Kohlberg's theory.

Jean Piaget was among the first to explore the ways individuals progress in applying reason and critical thinking over time. Kohlberg built on this idea to formulate his six stages of moral development. These stages were highly regarded in the 1970s. However, the fact that women repeatedly attained Stage 3 while men often attained Stages 4 and 5 prompted Gilligan to observe a problematic bias. In using only boys to validate his testing, Kohlberg limited the applicability of the test. In fact, his testing could not accurately assess girls' levels of moral development at all.

Gilligan's Stages of Moral Development

Using a three-stage model, Gilligan (1982) presented a process in which each woman's sense of self is recognized as a primary factor in decision-making. Each stage focuses on developmental hurdles and values inherent to that particular stage. The three stages as defined by Gilligan are as follows. The first stage is the pre-conventional stage. At this point, the young girl's moral focus is on the self and self-survival. Thus, practicality motivates decisions. The second stage, the conventional stage, is when a sense of responsibility to others develops. The ability to show kindness to others, including to the point of self-sacrifice, becomes important. Finally, during the third stage, the post-conventional stage, the woman realizes the importance of placing her needs at the same level of importance as the needs of others. The focus shifts from a woman receiving affirmation based on the perception of her as "good" to a woman realizing core human truths regarding the lack of ethics involved in human aggression and exploitation.

Subversive Nature of Theory

The era in the U.S. history in which Gilligan found herself, the 1960s, was the time of the anti-Vietnam war movement, civil rights movement, gay liberation movement, and the second wave of feminism women's movement. Through working closely with Kohlberg, and Erikson, both of whom ascribed to the works of Sigmund Freud and Jean Piaget, Gilligan saw how masculine qualities the standard by which women were measured. Studies of boys and men became and still are the standard for all of human development. This system depends upon women remaining silent, subordinate, and cooperative.

There were clear power differentials between Gilligan and Kohlberg. As his research assistant, Gilligan was bold and criticized his male-focused approach to the stages of moral development. She realized that the research methodology of the studies all of these men used to support their theories was flawed. The populations used in the study of human development were boys and men, only generalizable to half of the population and not applicable to females. Gilligans book *In a Different Voice* was published again in 2016. In it she writes about where women fit into the man's life cycle, concepts of self, morality, and what maturity looks like for women. Gilligan did not stay silent. She was powerful and uncooperative with the values and beliefs that did not fit for her, and she conducted research to demonstrate that women have a different model of human development than that of men.

This chapter on human growth and development has highlighted that what is often viewed by our society as applicable to humans in general, should be minimally viewed through a gendered lens. One size does not fit all, or rather one overarching theory of human growth and development based on studies with men, does not necessarily apply to women. As Maher, Ainsworth, and Gilligan have all demonstrated, women view the nature of self through relationships. Each of the women discussed in this chapter provided significant contributions to human growth and development. Each woman prioritized health and wellness, but did not agree on feminist ideals. Margaret Mahler, Mary Ainsworth, and Carol Gilligan contributed in significant ways to our conceptualization and understanding of human growth and development.

REFERENCES

Ainsworth, M. D. S (1983). Mary D. Salter Ainsworth. In A. N. 0'Connell & N. F. Russo (eds.), *Models of Achievement: Reflections of Eminent Women in Psychology* (pp. 200–219). New York: Columbia University Press.

Ainsworth, M. D. S., & Bell, S. M. (1970). Attachment, exploration, and separation: Illustrated by the behavior of one-year-olds in a strange situation. *Child Development*, *41*(1), 49–67. https://www.jstor.org/stable/1127388

Ainsworth, M. D., Blehar, M., Waters, E., & Wall, S. (1978). *Patterns of Attachment: A Psychological Study of the Strange Situation*. Erlbaum.

Ainsworth, M. D, & Wittig, B. (1969). Attachment and exploratory behavior of one-year-olds in a strange situation. In B. Foss (ed.), *Determinants of Infant Behavior* (Vol. IV, pp. 113–136). Methuen.

Bergman, A. (1999). *Ours, Yours, Mine: Mutuality and the Emergence of the Separate Self.* Jason Aronson.

Bihari, P. (2016). Aspects of anti-Semitism in Hungary, 1915–1918. *Quest: Issues in Contemporary Jewish History*, *9*, 58–93. http://www.quest-cdecjournal.it/focus.php?id=377

Blatz, W. (1940). *Hostages to Peace: Parents and the Children of Democracy*. Morrow.

Bowlby, J. (1958). The nature of the child's tie to his mother. *International Journal of Psychoanalysis*, *XXXIX*, 1–23. http://www.psychology.sunysb.edu/attachment/online/nature%20of%20the%20childs%20tie%20bowlby.pdf

Bowlby, J. (1959). Separation anxiety. *International Journal of Psychoanalysis*, *XLI*, 1–25. https://www.sas.upenn.edu/~cavitch/pdf-library/Bowlby_Separation.pdf

Bowlby, J. (1960). Grief and mourning in infancy and early childhood. *The Psychoanalytic Study of the Child*, *VX*, 3–39. doi:10.1080/00797308.1960.11822566

Bowlby, J., Ainsworth, M., Boston, M., & Rosenbluth, D. (1956). The effects of mother-child separation: A follow-up study. *British Journal of Medical Psychology*, *29*, 211–247. doi:10.1111/j.2044-8341.1956.tb00915.x

Bretherton, I. (1992). The origins of attachment theory: John Bowlby and Mary Ainsworth. *Developmental Psychology*, *28*(5), 759–775. doi:10.1037/0012-1649.28.5.759

Coates, S. (2004). John Bowlby and Margaret S. Mahler: Their lives and theories. *Journal of the American Psychoanalytic Association*, *52*(2), 571–601. doi:10.1177/00030651040520020601

Cox, S. M. (2006). Bridging attachment theory and attachment parenting with feminist methods of inquiry. *Journal of the Motherhood Initiative for Research and Community Involvement, 8*(1), 83–95. https://jarm.journals.yorku.ca/index.php/jarm/article/viewFile/5015/4209

Freud, Sigmund (1962). *Three Essays on the Theory of Sexuality* (J. Strachey, Trans.). Basic Books.

Gilligan, C. (1977). In a different voice: Women's conceptions of self and of morality. *Harvard Educational Review, 47*(4), 481–517. doi:10.17763/haer.47.4.g6167429416hg5l0

Gilligan, C. (1982). *In a Different Voice: Psychological Theory and Women's Development.* Harvard University Press. doi:10.17763/haer.47.4.g6167429416hg5l0

Gilligan, Carol. (2011). *Looking Back to Look Forward: Revisiting in a Different Voice*. Classics@ 9. Washington, DC: Center for Hellenic Studies. http://nrs.harvard.edu/urn-3:hlnc.essay:Gilligan.Looking_Back_to_Look_Forward.2011

Mahler, M. (1977). Psychoanalytic movement. Oral History Research Office, Columbia University.

Mahler, M. S. (1979). The selected papers of Margaret S. Mahler, M.D. The Selected Papers of Margaret S. Mahler, M.D.

Mahler, M. S., & Furer, M. (1960). Observations on research regarding the "symbiotic syndrome" of infantile psychosis. *The Psychoanalytic Quarterly, 29,* 317–327. doi:10.1080/21674086.1960.11926177

Mahler, S., Pine, M. M., & Bergman, A. (1973). *The Psychological Birth of the Human Infant.* Basic Books.

Main, M., & Solomon, J. (1986). Discovery of a new, insecure-disorganized/disoriented attachment pattern. In M. Yogman & T. B. Brazelton (eds.), *Affective Development in Infancy* (pp. 95–124). Ablex.

Medea, A. (March 1, 2009). Carol Gilligan. Jewish Women's Archive. https://jwa.org/encyclopedia/article/gilligan-carol

Pauley, B. F. (1992). *From Prejudice to Persecution: A History of Austrian Anti-Semitism.* University of North Carolina Press.

Stepansky, P. E. (1988). *The Memoirs of Margaret S. Mahler.* Free Press.

Woods, C. J. (1996). Gender differences in moral development and acquisition: A review of Kohlberg's and Gilligan's models of justice and care. *Social Behavior and Personality: An International Journal, 24*, 375–384. doi:10.2224/sbp.1996.24.4.375

Chapter 2

Psychodynamic Theorists

Foundational to the practice of counseling and psychotherapy are psychodynamic theories and psychoanalysis, whose underlying premises and concepts still influence many contemporary theories. Each theory born after psychoanalysis either modified concepts or diverged in conception and practice. Psychodynamic theories focus on the role of the unconscious in the manifestation of behavior and personality. The roles of anxiety and instinctual drives are given special attention as influential factors stemming from the depths of the unconscious. Many childhood and human developmental theories have emerged from the foundation of psychodynamic concepts.

As mentioned in chapter 1, many of these theories have been expanded or modified to include more contemporary, multicultural, and pluralistic perspectives. While Sigmund Freud (1856–1939) is the thinker most widely credited with the development of this theory, women have modified and expanded upon psychodynamic theories in important ways. Sigmund Freud's daughter Anna Freud (1895–1982) was an Austrian psychoanalyst who contributed significantly to the field of psychoanalysis. Along with Anna Freud, Melanie Klein (1882–1960) is credited with applying psychoanalytic concepts to working with children. Both women are associated with the origins of psychoanalytic child psychology. Karen Horney (1885–1952) was a German-born psychoanalyst whose voice diverged from Freud's. Her perspective regarding some of Freud's concepts, especially sexuality and instinctual drives, varied from Freud's traditional male-centered views.

THEORIST BIOGRAPHIES: ANNA FREUD AND MELANIE KLEIN

Anna Freud and Melanie Klein are both credited with the establishment of child analysis, a field which is based upon the psychoanalytic tradition. Both women were heavily influenced by Sigmund Freud's ideas and teachings. However, each woman responded to this knowledge in different ways, ultimately leading to the expansion and establishment of two separate theories. The two theories that were eventually born through the theorists became significant forces in the psychoanalytic field. Viner (1996) described both theories as valid alternative theories. Anna Freud's ideas led to the development of ego psychology, and Melanie Klein's work led to the theory of object relations, both of which subsequently impacted much of the developmental literature on attachment and parenting. The evolution of each remarkable woman is explained parallel to her developed theory. Key concepts from each theory are presented. Special attention is given to the ways in which the two theories diverge conceptually and practically.

Anna Freud was born in winter 1895 in Vienna and lived until fall 1982, when she passed away in London at the age of eighty-six. Freud was a sensitive child who eventually matured into a young woman who refused to comply with gendered and societal expectations and invaluably contributed to the field of psychoanalysis (Gurfinkel, 2016; Solnit, 1997). The daughter of Sigmund Freud, Anna Freud was certainly influenced by her father, yet much of her work represents a revision of his thoughts and ideas, especially in their application to children. Freud began her professional life as an educator, but in the early 1920s she was compelled to enter the world of psychoanalysis with the intent to apply it to children in need in both educational and clinical settings (Viner, 1996). Freud quickly gained traction in the Vienna Psychoanalytic Society and went on to publish her first book, *An Introduction to the Technique of Child Analysis*, in 1927. She later extended her father's ideas on the function of the ego, publishing *The Ego and the Mechanisms of Defense* in 1936. This work made her even more indispensable in psychoanalytic societies. Freud presented to her father on his eightieth birthday (Solnit, 1997).

Freud was able to move between theory and practice throughout her professional career. She founded nurseries for children displaced by World War II in Vienna and London, where she both observed and worked with children. From these observations and practices, Freud developed advanced theoretical insight into child development that extended her father's concept of psychosexual stages. She applied her modified version of psychoanalysis to these cases, highlighting the need for appropriate developmental considerations (Solnit, 1997). Freud was truly a "champion for war torn families at the time of the Second World War . . . she inspired her communities to rise their obligations" (Cheifetz, 2014, p. 226). With her lifelong companion and partner, Dorothy Burlingham, Freud co-founded the Hempstead War Nurseries (1940s) and Hempstead Center (1950s) to continue working with children affected by war (Ludwig-Körner, 2017; Young-Bruehl, 2004).

Melanie Klein was born Melanie Reizes in Vienna in the spring of 1882 and passed away in London during fall 1960 at the age of seventy-eight. Her entrance into and passage through life paralleled those of Anna Freud, yet the two theorists differed in their interpretation and application of child psychoanalysis. Klein married Arthur Klein at the age of twenty-one and was the mother of three children, Klein first became interested in psychoanalysis when considering herself and her children. Klein had a complex and strained relationship with her mother, an aspect of her life that may well be reflected in her theoretical conceptions. In 1919, after presenting her own theoretical analysis and initial ideas, she entered the Hungarian Psychoanalytic Society. Her first published work, *The Development of the Child* (1923), was well received (Donaldson, 1996).

In the early 1920s, Klein's marriage dissolved, and she moved to Berlin to begin constructing her play technique and theoretical concepts regarding children's unconscious existence and experience. Klein's remarkable technique was applied to children as young as two years old. Her ability to analyze and interpret children's play was both impressive and provocative (Proner, 1998). Klein found her home in London in 1926, where she further established herself in the British Psychoanalytic Society and came head to head with Anna Freud (Viner, 1996).

Key Concepts and Utilization of Theory

Anna Freud and Melanie Klein's divergence in their theoretical ideas began in the 1920s, when their disagreements with and challenges of one another's positions were made public in various outlets. The hostility generated by the theorists' contrasting views of child analysis culminated in the widely publicized exchanges known as the controversial discussions (CDs), which took place between 1942 and 1944. According to Shapira (2017), "The CDs are often seen by psychoanalysts as a metaphorical war between Sigmund Freud's 'two daughters'—one of them his biological daughter and the other a potential intellectual heir—fighting over who would continue the work of psychoanalysis" (p. 174). The result of these CDs was the splitting of the field into Anna Freud's ideas, which led to ego psychology, and Melanie Klein's ideas, which led to object relations theory (Donaldson, 1996; Shapira, 2017). Both schools of thought offered valid, alternative theories of psychoanalysis (Viner, 1996). The major distinctions between the Freudian and Kleinian schools of child analysis are highlighted later in this chapter (figure 1).

Anna Freud's primary focus was utilizing her theoretical insight to develop "practical applications which would enhance the child's conditions for optimal development" (Tischler, 2014, p. 156). She emphasized the importance of looking at the whole child and taking both internal and external experiences into account. She is well known for the concept of *developmental lines* (Tischler, 2014). *Developmental lines* present the developmental stages as the building blocks of the child's overall systemic development. When a practitioner views a child's development across each line, a clearer picture emerges. Murray Harrison (2013) noted that "Anna Freud attempted to integrate the child development she was learning from her observation of children, with her father's psychoanalytic theory. . . . [Her] theoretical model of *developmental lines* represented a major contribution in attempt to capture the complexity of development" (p. 324). Freud understood that a disturbance in one line, or area of development, influenced the whole of development. The six lines of development are as follows:

1. Dependency to emotional regulation, wherein the child can overcome infantile struggles and projections and transfer intimacy to outside the family.
2. Suckling to rational eating.
3. Use of diapers to control of bladder and bowels.
4. Irresponsible to responsible management of the body.
5. Ego-centrism to reciprocal relationships with peers.
6. Ability to achieve both play and work (Solnit, 1997; Tischler, 2014).

Through her extensive observations and clinical experiences, Freud found that normal versus pathological development was dependent on the following four factors: that the experience of the child does not depart drastically from the norm; that internally, the child's personality matures at about the same rate as other children's personalities; that if intervention is needed, it is well timed; and finally, that the child's developing ego is able to make age-appropriate compromises or adequate defenses (Solnit, 1997).

Murray Harrison (2013) applied Freud's conceptual framework of *developmental lines* to a set of interventions called *developmental help*. *Developmental help* can be used as a therapeutic intervention with children who have not benefited from the normal experience of the four aforementioned factors. *Developmental help* encompasses the following: promoting positive interactions, addressing primitive defenses, containing transference, giving meaning to thoughts and actions by providing terminology to describe mental states, and helping the child to differentiate between cause and effect. Practically speaking, *developmental help* involves focusing on the therapeutic relationship and building rapport with child, giving words to the child's sense and understanding of experience, helping the child to regulate emotions (containment), and facilitating the building of new competencies toward development (Murray Harrison, 2013). Murray Harrison (2013) considered the relationship between the analyst and the child to be comparable to that of the "caregiving relationship" (p. 326). This application of Anna Freud's work in the conceptualization of *developmental help* further differentiates her theory from classical psychoanalysis given the focus and significance of the therapeutic relationship.

Melanie Klein viewed the infant and young child as no one before her had. She was truly a pioneer in applying psychoanalytic principles to the infant psyche (Hindle, 2017). Klein's compassion for the infant's struggles is noteworthy. Hindle (2017) stated,

> What comes across in the numerous quotes from Klein's personal papers as well as her published work, is her sensitivity and compassion for the plight of young children and their often silent-suffering—a factor that any child psychotherapists or others can relate to. (p. 90)

Klein presented a method she referred to as *Kinderanalyse*, which was a simple yet powerful expansion of traditional adult psychoanalysis. Klein viewed the early development of the superego as severe and blamed much of the child's anxiety and resulting fear and hostility on the young superego. This hostility and aggression were most often projected onto the child's love object, or in early childhood, the primary caregiver. The aim of therapy was to decrease and manage the child's anxiety as a result of the "severity of the early superego" (Donaldson, 1996, p. 166).

Klein saw children's play as the gateway to understanding their unconscious. She, therefore, developed the *play technique* to facilitate the discovery of unconscious motives and desires. The *play technique* stresses the following when a therapist is setting up therapy with a young child: a conducive setting for the child to explore, the use of play objects, role-playing, games suited for children, and limit-setting. Klein stressed the significance of observing the child's play sequence and associated emotions that might give insight into underlying unconscious anxieties (Hindle, 2017). Through this *play technique*, the earliest form of play therapy was born. Klein believed that children were capable of much more insight than one might expect, and she maintained the importance of applying the transference relationship and associated interpretation directly to a child. Klein believed that as a child's form of free association, play is particularly effective because of "the closer connection between the conscious and unconscious in young children" (Donaldson, 1996, p. 6).

As innovative and revolutionary as Klein's ideas were, they were often met with objection and seen as controversial. Simply put, many fellow analysts found the ideas of infant aggression, sexuality, and sadism to be shocking and frightening to conceptualize. Proner (1998) stated, "Her understanding seemed to grasp the bodily essence of human beginnings and penetrate and disturb our equilibrium. Klein brings us right inside our own sensate parts. She draws us close to our infantile selves, makes us fascinated but then shocks, frightens, and excited us with the sexuality and brutality" (p. 452). Klein fully immersed herself in the young child's experience, resulting in her ideas regarding *projective identification*. Projective identification refers to the idea that children not only project their fear and aggression on to their love object(s), but they also internalize these feelings. These Kleinian conceptualizations eventually led to the branch of psychoanalytic theory known as object relations theory, which continues the conceptual and practical application of this line of thinking (Donaldson, 1996; Proner, 1998). Klein maintained that the process of change and healing occurs in the same place from which aggression and hostility spring because even among the darkest parts of the psyche, there is love. Through a contained analytic stance on the part of the therapist, the child can recover "the internal parts of the self—lost through projection onto others" (Proner, 1998, p. 455). Klein emphasized that this is a gradual process that entails the "returning of projections and undoing of splits" (p. 455). When the child experiences the loving impulses that are present within, the child is able to combat the negative impulses.

While Freud and Klein shared the conceptual basis of psychoanalytic theory, they diverged significantly in their views on the nature of the child's mind and the application of psychoanalysis to children (Viner, 1996). According to Viner (1996), the theorists' "fundamentally opposed concepts of the strength of the superego in small children led to the emergence of contradictory techniques in almost all elements of the analysis of children" (p. 7). Table 2.1 illustrates the theorists' respective positions.

The major differences between Anna Freud's and Melanie Klein's perspectives on child analysis are as follows:

Subversive Nature of Theories

In describing the burden and foremost the legacy of Anna Freud, Ignatieff (1988) said, "She was his dutiful daughter, . . . the one who found her destiny safeguarding the shrine of his achievement . . . nevertheless she managed her escape, becoming both a theoretical innovator and a woman in her own right. She inherited the mantle, yet she survived the weight" (as cited in Tischler, 2014, p. 157). Anna Freud expanded upon and augmented her father's ideas; she was not crushed by the weight of this mantle. In some respects, Freud challenged her father's original thoughts. Cohler and Galatzer-Levy (2008) noted, "Many of Anna Freud's most important contributions involved rejection of her father's ideas" (p. 17). Anna Freud focused on the power of the

Table 2.1 Differences between Theoretical Positions of Freud and Klein (Donaldson, 1996; Roazen, 1991; Shapira, 2017; Tischler, 2014; Viner, 1996)

Freud	*Klein*
Analyst should create a relationship with the child before commencing analysis (conscious cooperation from child)	Analyst should take a classic psychoanalyst stance in order to provoke transference (unconscious cooperation).
Because children are too young to be analyzed in the traditional Freudian manner, their dreams are analyzed	Children's unconscious is analyzed through play and nonverbal behavior
Children's sense of good and bad does not develop until the phallic stage	Children's sense of good and bad develops in the earlier oral stage
	Children do not need therapy unless they are acting out vs. all children can be analyzed
Therapy for children can be applied in educational settings and teachers and social workers can adapt and use it in these settings	Therapy is based in clinical settings and best done by classically trained psychoanalysts
Parents are asked to be active supports in the process of therapy	Parents are unnecessary in the process of therapy
Children do not remember trauma like adults do, and they must have their ego built up before they can be analyzed as adults would; therefore, the focus of therapy is building up the ego	Children can be viewed as miniature adults and can be analyzed in similar ways as adults
When the child's superego develops, the sexual energy projected on to parents is resolved	The superego develops in infancy and is the reason for the fear and aggression seen in infants
Anna Freud's theory led to an advanced understanding of child development	Melanie Klein's theory became the earliest form of play therapy

ego and associated defenses rather than the drive theory established by her father. She also demonstrated through years of careful, direct observation how fruitful the methodology could be even though her father had previously undervalued it. Additionally, by focusing on developmental lines, she showcased the importance of interactional factors and their impact on development rather than the previously integrated psychosexual stages presented by her father (Cohler & Galatzer-Levy, 2008).

Anna Freud stressed the importance of social factors to individual development. She also emphasized the importance of focusing on the individual's entire lifespan and the corresponding series of developmental events rather than one point in life, such as early childhood. Midgley (2012) stated that Freud was remarkable in that she focused on the humanizing process, the normal development that humans may experience rather than just psychopathology. This contrasted with the theoretical outlook of the time. Freud believed that there were multiple causes of psychopathology and was not as reductionistic or deterministic as her father. Along with more traditional utilizations of research, Freud emphasized the importance of observations through action research and became noteworthy as an innovator in the field (Ludwig-Körner, 2017). According to Young-Bruehl (2004), "As a researcher Anna Freud was certainly the great model, first in the 1930s, then as the codirector with Dorothy Burlingham of the Hempstead War Nurseries in the 1940s, later the cofounder in the 1950s of the Hempstead Center, which was for decades the most important psychoanalytic research center in the world" (p. 195). Freud and Burlingham quietly but assuredly impacted the field of child development by applying both observational and clinical data to theory and practice in a variety of altruistic endeavors. Both personally and professionally, Freud can be viewed as subversive. "Calmly refusing to comply with gender expectations" (Gurfinkel, 2016, p. 295), Freud chose a life that was different from the lives of many of the women of her time. In the 1920s, she found her "helpmate and essential other" (Cohler & Galatzer-Levy, 2008, p. 17) in Dorothy Burlingham, and the two women remained connected both personally and professionally for the remainder of their lives. Young-Bruehl (2004) elaborated on Freud's legacy by saying that she had contributed to the welfare of children worldwide. Solnit (1997) succinctly stated that our dept to Anna Freud is incalculable.

Melanie Klein's work, although based largely on Sigmund Freud's theory, departed in significant ways. Klein believed that libidinal stages are present from birth and, therefore, must be attended to during child analysis. In other words, the superego is present from birth; it does not form as a result of the Oedipus complex as Sigmund Freud believed (Donaldson, 1996). The existence of the superego from infancy is the cause of infant anxiety, and this anxiety must be identified and managed by the analyst during the child's treatment. With the exception of Little Hans in 1909, Sigmund Freud's work largely focused on adults. Klein established her niche by concentrating on the missed opportunity of delving into the infant's unconscious world after she theorized the chaotic nature of its existence (Decker, 1990; Viner, 1996). Furthermore, while Sigmund Freud's focus was primarily on the father and the impact of the relationship resulting from that line of care, Klein's work led to a focus on the mother-child relationship and the resulting development, whether healthy or unhealthy (Decker, 1990).

Throughout her professional career, Klein often faced criticism for her ideas. Generally speaking, "it was the male analysts who attacked Klein's ideas, while the female analysts, including Karen Horney, were more receptive" (Donaldson, 1996, p. 164). (This was, of course, with the exception of Anna Freud.) Klein was a divorced woman who did not have any formal college education in a field dominated by men. Her ideas prevailed despite this. Proner (1998) noted that "as a professional figure, Klein represents the wounded healer, a source of inspiration and renewal for professional work and life" (p. 455). Klein's persistence and perseverance in the face of adversity and intense criticism led to the staying power of her theory and ideas. Her legacy is a remarkable and admirable one.

THEORIST BIOGRAPHY: KAREN HORNEY

Karen Horney was born Karen Danielsen in 1885 in Germany and passed away in 1952 in New York City at the age of sixty-seven. Horney was formally educated as a medical doctor, but she eventually found her way to the Berlin Psychoanalytic Institute where she became an instructor and researcher. She married Oskar Horney in 1906 and had three daughters. Horney separated from her husband in 1926, and they divorced in 1937 (Quinn, 2019).

Key Concepts and Utilization of Theory

In 1932, she fled to the United States from Europe and took up residence at the Chicago Institute for Psychoanalysis, where she later became the associate director. After another move in the States, Horney established herself in the New York Psychoanalytic Institute where she continued developing her theory. Horney's theory stood in contrast to Freud's view of penis envy and his focus on male biology and superiority. Within the field of psychoanalysis, she became associated with neo-Freudianism, also referred to as psychodynamic psychiatry (Ingram, 2012). Trahair (1989) argued that "she used psychoanalysis, rebelled against it, challenged the patriarchal ideology in Freud's ideas including the narrow range of his therapeutic practices, and questioned the oppressive conventions attached both to marriage in her youth and the infantile interest in women's bodies that takes hold in adult life" (p. 196). Horney essentially became the first feminist psychotherapist, and when she died in the 1950s, she left behind a far-reaching legacy. Her theoretical ideas led to the genesis of yet another branch of psychoanalysis through the eventual development of interpersonal theory (Ortmeyer, 1995).

Feminist underpinnings and interpretations. Horney certainly traveled where no man had gone before. Patey (1987) noted, "What *do* women want? Sigmund Freud was never able to satisfactorily answer that question. His failure to provide an acceptable interpretation of the female psyche has left psychoanalysis disfavored by contemporary feminists" (p. 456). Horney's success in building a theory of female psychology from the psychoanalytic bedrock is indeed impressive and significant. Horney's writings led to the conclusion that women's neuroses are the product of living in a patriarchal society. In order to overcome the devaluing and exploitive nature and influence of culture and society, one must first understand it (Patey, 1987;

Trahair, 1989). Growing up female in our society is growing up neurotic, given how women are objectified, devalued, and placed in a position of powerless responsibility. Women project images of themselves as *ideal selves* (dictated by society) that are constraining and impossible to achieve. When the ideal self is recognized and challenged, an *authentic self* can be constructed through a genuine reflection of internal worth, experience, and value (Patey, 1987).

Theoretical constructs. Horney developed her theory of neurosis to aid in explaining the symptomology of women and culture and society's impact on them. In addition to deconstructing that impact, she considered the home environment where "the cultural conflict can be experienced more intensely if the home presents similar unresolved conflicts if parenting is inadequate" (Patey, 1987, p. 458). Horney's theory of child development has humanistic as well as feminist underpinnings, in that she believed that the child's *authentic self* would naturally emerge if allowed to grow unimpeded. When children are raised with empathy, warmth, respect, and validation, they develop a sense of *we-ness* in their relationships with their primary caregivers. This type of relationship promotes a sense of belonging, which in turn instills in the children *basic confidence* in their self-worth and value as human beings.

Horney identified five characteristics of healthy self-development, which are indicative of the identification of the *authentic self.* First, the child can be *spontaneous* and is able to act on their needs and desires. Second, they can enjoy themselves in their experiences through *imagination and creativity.* Third, they can recognize their *limitations* and boundaries within this authentic enjoyment of themselves. Fourth, they can recognize their own growth and developmental evolution, as they gain a sense of *identity.* Lastly, self-realizing children can *accurately assess* their environments and themselves, thus living in truth (DeRobertis, 2006). While adequate parental love and bonds facilitate healthy self-development, inadequate parenting may result in the opposite. Children from tumultuous home environments may never develop *basic confidence* and instead come to develop *basic anxiety.* A lack of parental warmth, respect, and love leads children to feel alone and vulnerable, preventing them from developing the confidence they need to be who they are. According to DeRobertis (2006), "In other words, if being themselves arouses basic anxiety, then the only viable alternative to quell their fears of abandonment is to avoid the real self" (p. 187).

Horney identified three ways of being that are constructed in individuals who have abandoned the *authentic self* for *interpersonal moves* that help them avoid fundamental insecurity (*basic anxiety*). These three ways of being and responses to childhood anxiety are "the dependent, the domineering, and the detached type," they manifest in *interpersonal moves* that are characterized by *moving toward, moving against, or moving away* from others, respectively (DeRobertis, 2006; Ingram, 2012; Patey, 1987, p. 458). Horney saw that women predominantly chose their *interpersonal move* to be the dependent, or the *moving toward*, constructed personality. The process of change in therapy, therefore, first requires acknowledging the loss of the *authentic self* due to both culture and environment; it then requires working through the resulting repressed rage and dependency that this early loss fostered. In therapy, "the woman has nothing to lose and everything to gain the realization of her authentic self" (Patey, 1987, p. 459). The final move one makes over the course of successful treatment is from "feminine type" to "female hero" (p. 459).

Subversive Nature of Theory

Karen Horney also courageously raised her voice against Freud's at a time when that kind of divergent thinking was met with opposition. DeRobertis (2006) stated that "Horney rejected the reductionistic, mechanistic view of the mind that Freud espoused" (p. 183). As a neo-Freudian, Horney incorporated the first feminist and humanistic influences into a deterministic framework and pushed back on the Freudian doctrine of the time. Horney went on to develop a theory that more accurately portrayed and depicted women's lives and experiences, especially as situated in the early to mid-1900s. Horney was a revolutionary woman and thinker, giving voice to the plight of women that had been so obviously overlooked and undervalued. Patey (1987) wrote, "She lived the conflict described in her work: the desire for love and acceptance versus the need to oppose the values that define lovability and acceptability in our society. It took great courage to challenge the prevalent mode of thought in a male-dominated field such as psychoanalysis, and she had much rigorous opposition" (p. 456).

In 1941, Horney split from the New York Psychoanalytic Institute as a result of her ideas diverging so dramatically from Freud's. Members of this society launched a campaign against her in response to the chaos that ensued because of her departure. Despite this, her voice and ideas have remained. According to Quinn (2019),

> Fortunately, Karen Horney's writings have saved her from the oblivion to which some of her enemies tried to consign her. Far from being trivial or unimportant, Horney was the first, and perhaps the best, critic of Freud's ideas about women. (p. 2)

Horney innately knew in the 1920s what feminist and postmodern thinkers would only eventually come to write about in the 1970s. She was truly a woman ahead of her time, and her legacy inspired so many who came after her (Quinn, 2019). Her independent mind, tenacity of spirit, and devotion to her own truth of experience ensured that her voice would not go unheard. Her voice still echoes today in the lasting impact she made on psychoanalytic and psychodynamic theories.

The three women covered in this chapter, Freud, Klein, and Horney each impacted the field of counseling and psychotherapy. Specifically, each woman was trained in psychodynamic theory and yet diverged from completely embracing all of the tenets and thoughts of Sigmund Freud in significant ways. Each woman experienced resistance to her thoughts and ideas, yet persevered with courage and a conviction in their theoretical perspectives. Without the contributions of these three women, psychodynamic theory would have maintained its singular perspective and Eurocentric application in a world that is full of diversity of culture, gender, and thoughts.

REFERENCES

Cheifetz, P. (2014). [Review of the book *Reading Anna Freud* by Nick Midgley]. *Journal of the Canadian Academy of Child & Adolescent Psychiatry*, *23*(3), 226. https://www.ncbi.nlm.nih.gov/pmc/articles/PMC4197523/pdf/ccap-23-226.pdf

Cohler, B., & Galatzer-Levy, R. (2008). Freud, Anna, and the problem of female sexuality. *Psychoanalytic Inquiry*, *28*(1), 3–26. doi:10.1080/07351690701787085

Decker, H. S. (1990). [Review of the book *Reshaping the Psychoanalytic Domain: The Work of Melanie Klein, W. R. D. Fairbain, and D. W. Winnicott* by Judith M. Hughes]. *American Historical Review*, *95*(4), 1153–1154. doi:10.1086/ahr/95.4.1153-a

DeRobertis, E. M. (2006). Deriving a humanistic theory of child development from the works of Carl R. Rogers and Karen Horney. *Humanistic Psychologist*, *34*(2), 177–199. doi:10.1207/s15473333thp3402_5

Donaldson, G. (1996). Between practice and theory: Melanie Klein, Anna Freud and the development of child analysis. *Journal of the History of the Behavioral Sciences*, *32*(2), 160–176. doi:10.1002/(SICI)1520-6696(199604)32:2%3C160::AID-JHBS4%3E3.0.CO;2-%23

Gurfinkel, H. (2016). The case history of Anna Freud. *Papers on Language & Literature*, *52*(3), 295–298. https://www.questia.com/library/journal/1G1-462787955/the-case-history-of-anna-freud

Hindle, D. (2017). Melanie Klein revisited. *Infant Observation*, *20*(1), 89–93.

Ingram, D. H. (2012). Who was Karen Horney? *Psychiatric Times*, *29*(3), 22–23. https://www.psychiatrictimes.com/view/who-was-karen-horney

Ludwig-Körner, C. (2017). Anna Freud and observation: Memoirs of her colleagues from the Hampstead war nurseries. *Journal of Infant, Child & Adolescent Psychotherapy*, *16*(2), 131–137. doi:10.1080/15289168.2017.1307072

Midgley, N. (2012). The course of life: A 1979 lecture by Anna Freud. *British Journal of Psychotherapy*, *28*(3), 395–399. doi:10.1111/j.1752-0118.2012.01305.x

Murray Harrison, A. (2013). Comments on: "Developmental Psychoanalysis and Developmental Objects." *Psychoanalytic Inquiry*, *33*(4), 323–329. doi:10.1080/07351690.2013.803345

Ortmeyer, D. (1995). History of the founders of interpersonal psychoanalysis. In M. Lionells, J. Fiscalini, C.H. Mann, & D. B. Stern (eds.), *Handbook of Interpersonal Psychoanalysis* (pp. 3–27).

Patey, H. (1987). [Review of the book *The Feminist Legacy of Karen Horney* by Marcia Westkott]. *Canadian Journal of Women & the Law*, 2(2), 455–459.

Proner, K. (1998). Learning and teaching the theories of Melanie Klein. *Journal of Child Psychotherapy*, *24*(3), 449–460. doi:10.1080/00754179808414830

Quinn, S. (2019). *A Mind of Her Own: The Life of Karen Horney*. Plunkett Lake Press.

Roazen, P. (1991). [Review of the book *The Technique of Child Analysis: Discussions with Anna Freud* by Joseph Sandier, Hansi Kennedy, and Robert L. Tyson]. *Journal of the History of the Behavioral Sciences*, *27*(3), 281–283. doi:10.1002/1520-6696(199107)27:3<281::AID-JHBS2300270330>3.0.CO;2-N

Shapira, M. (2017). Interpersonal rivalries, gender and the intellectual and scientific making of psychoanalysis in 1940s Britain. *History of Psychology*, *20*(2), 172–194. https://psycnet.apa.org/doi/10.1037/hop0000056

Solnit, A. J. (1997). A legacy: Anna Freud's views on childhood and development. *Child Psychiatry & Human Development*, *28*(1), 5–14. doi:10.1023/A:1025136817483

Tischler, L. (2014). Anna Freud: A new look at development. *British Journal of Psychotherapy*, *30*(2), 154–168. doi:10.1111/bjp.1208

Trahair, R. (1989). [Review of the book *The Feminist Legacy of Karen Horney* by Marcia Westkott]. *Journal of the History of the Behavioral Sciences*, *25*(2), 196–198. doi:10.1002/1520-6696(198904)25:2<196::AID-JHBS2300250221>3.0.CO;2-O

Viner, R. (1996). Melanie Klein and Anna Freud: The discourse of the early dispute. *Journal of the History of the Behavioral Sciences*, *32*(1), 4–15. doi:10.1002/(SICI)1520-6696(199601)32:1<4::AID-JHBS1>3.0.CO;2-Y

Young-Bruehl, E. (2004). Anna Freud and Dorothy Burlingham at Hempstead: The origins of psychoanalytic parent-infant observation. *Annual of Psychoanalysis*, *32*, 185–197. https://www.pep-web.org/document.php?id=aop.032.0185a

Chapter 3

Humanistic Theorists

Humanism emerged in response to psychoanalysis, offering a fundamentally different view of human nature. Humanism focuses on the growth and potential of the human condition rather than reductionist, deterministic, and instinctual conceptualizations. Accordingly, humans are considered to be self-aware, self-directed, conscientious, and, therefore, optimistic regarding their existence. The focus of humanistic theories is relational. Practitioners encounter their clients through meaningful psychological contact, which promotes awareness, growth, and potential. Carl Rogers became known for his humanistic approach and in particular, the development of person-centered theory. Rogers's daughter, Natalie Rogers (1928–2015), made her own name in the humanistic movement by establishing person-centered expressive arts therapy. Natalie Rogers focused on the power of human potential via connection and creativity through the modality of expressive arts. Existential and Gestalt theories also emerged as part of the humanistic theoretical movement. Fritz Perls is credited with the creation of Gestalt theory, yet his wife, Laura Perls (1905–1990), made significant contributions to this theory. A German-born psychologist, Perls became quite influential in the establishment and growth of Gestalt ideas in the United States. When her husband left his family to travel abroad and profess his theory, Perls stayed in the United States to nurture and develop Gestalt theory into what it is today.

THEORIST BIOGRAPHY: NATALIE ROGERS

Natalie Rogers was born in fall 1928 and passed away in fall 2015 at the age of eighty-seven. She was born to Carl and Helen Rogers in Rochester, New York, and at the age of twelve moved to Columbus, Ohio. Rogers was a devoted practitioner, theorist, activist, feminist, and teacher. Rogers married Lawrence H. Fuchs at the age of twenty-one and raised three daughters. Toward the middle of her life and following their divorce in 1970, she was compelled to cultivate an identity of her own, separate from the role of the traditional homemaker and wife that was common during the mid-1900s.

Key Concepts and Utilization of Theory

Her book *Emerging Woman* (1980) captured this transition "from a life defined by the expectations and needs of others to one that sprang from her own deep interiority. Hers was the voice of a generation of women who grew up in the claustrophobic 1950s who were expected to submerge their own potential in favor of their husbands" (O'Hara, 2016, p. 516). Rogers went on to create person-centered expressive arts therapy (PCEAT), which is based on PCA but promotes deeper exploration through expressive art mediums. She later published *The Creative Connection* (1993), which highlights the role of creativity in the therapeutic process. Rogers spent her final years in the San Francisco Bay Area, where she established the Person-Centered Expressive Therapy Institute (Anthony, 2015; Merry, 1997; O'Hara, 2016). Carl Rogers joined her in California during his last years, and together they facilitated workshops in university settings that promoted the person-centered approach (PCA; Sommers-Flanagan, 2007). Rogers was truly a humanistic pioneer, expanding and applying her father's work through her "fierce yet graceful efforts on behalf of people oppressed, peace, and the environment" (O'Hara, 2016, p. 561).

The work of Natalie Rogers led to what is currently known as expressive arts therapy. She gave concrete form to the concept of *creativity* through her extensive clinical work and writings on this cornerstone principle of her theory. Initially drawn to play therapy with children, Rogers found that applying various expressive media to her work with adult clients had a very powerful and profound effect (Sommers-Flanagan, 2007). Within a supportive, nonjudgmental, growth-promoting setting (using the core conditions of PCA), Rogers invited clients to express their inner emotions through "movement, drawing, painting, sculpting, music, writing, sound and improvisation" (Merry, 1997, p. 266). She was not concerned with the aesthetic or external value of the product; rather, she directed her clients' attention to the process of creation and the associated emotions that were accessed and released through that process. Rogers believed that by engaging in this process of creation within a safe, supportive environment, clients would be able to peel back layers of their defenses and begin the process of healing.

The process of change is evoked through what Rogers termed the *creative connection.* During an interview in 1997, she spoke of this process, noting,

"I realized that one expressive art form stimulates and nurtures another art form, evoking our inner truths which are often revealed with new depths and meaning. Inner healing was taking place" (Merry, 1997, p. 267). In other words, Rogers found that when her clients began to move or dance and follow that with art, the *sequence* of expression was extended and deepened. Clients achieved deeper insight and meaning. These deeper meanings were never analyzed or interpreted by Rogers but came forth from the clients during the process of creation. She viewed herself as a companion on their journey. Her role was to understand a client's view of the world while creating a safe and supportive environment for expression (Rogers et al., 2012).

Rogers also emphasized and expanded upon the concept of *fluidity*, which her father had introduced. Rogers viewed *fluidity* as an openness to experience that is ultimately connected with humans' tendency to actualize (Rogers et al., 2012). Sommers-Flanagan (2007) succinctly stated, "It is the failure to learn from experience that best characterizes psychopathology. Therefore, person-centered therapists work so hard to help clients become more open to learning from new experiences. This is also why rigidity is considered the antithesis of psychological health" (p. 124). Rogers's intention behind using expressive media was to break through barriers of self-imposed rigidity that blocked her clients from experience and learning. This rigidity ultimately caused suffering and prevented growth. By offering "stimulating and challenging experiences" (Rogers et al., 2012, p. 35), PCEAT aimed to reconnect clients to what they had blocked from themselves and from others. As a result, clients were free to *release their potential* and move toward wholeness and actualization.

Rogers found that utilizing expressive art media moves clients through the world of their emotions, allows them access to the unconscious, and may lead them to a place of deeper, more profound understanding regarding themselves, their spiritual nature, and their connection to the world. A further application of Rogers's work can be found in her emphasis on community-building and efforts toward envisioning peace. Rogers believed that "creativity overrides conformity and self-empowerment prepares us for action" (Rogers et al., 2012, p. 44). Once clients have connected to their own internal systems of healing and peace, they are empowered to connect to others and promote that peace externally. Rogers lived that example. Her own process of self-discovery and healing allowed her to extend healing and advocacy toward others and the greater world. She stated,

> If humanity was my client, I would do my best to open my heart to listen and to understand their terrible suffering, the injustices, the outrage. I believe the terrorist acts that are happening have root causes of oppression, poverty and a sense of hopelessness by those who commit them. . . . We would need to address

> ways to shift those root causes so that justice and a basic level of health and wellbeing were achieved. (Rogers et al., 2012, p. 45)

Rogers inspired many with her focus on social justice, advocacy, and peace. She felt an innate connection to the world and to humanity, and she believed that therapy should include that extension to the world outside.

Subversive Nature of Theory

Rogers was often compared to her father, and in many ways, she continued and expanded upon his work. However, she applied the ever-important concept of *fluidity,* which is a personality change process from rigidity to an openness to experiences. She was sometimes critiqued for being directive in a type of therapy recognized as nondirective (Anthony, 2015). Rogers balked at that critique. She insisted that she offered art media as another means of expression, and although this was a departure from how her father worked, "we are setting up a structure to allow people to have an experience, we're not directing the experience" (Rogers et al., 2012, p. 41). That experience was that which took place through the medium of art. She continued, saying, "It seems so difficult for some people to realize that offering an open-ended structure so that people can have a creative experience is not directing their outcome" (Rogers et al., 2012, p. 40). The result of Roger's insistence that structure was necessary to facilitate creativity affected subsequent theoretical developments and changed how theorists think about the role of structure in counseling and psychotherapy.

Furthermore, Rogers refused to justify her work in terms of her father's. She fully believed that Carl Rogers would have acknowledged the need for the continued development of the field and the theory and that he would have honored her response to experience, as revealed in the concept of *fluidity*. However, Rogers herself was more concerned with the effectiveness of her therapy and the successful transition to healing that PCEAT facilitated in so many individuals. She also focused on the application of her theory to power, privilege, and politics. Prior to Rogers, few therapists had focused on these systems of oppression. It may have been that Rogers was more attuned to this when others were overlooking it because she was a woman living during the second-wave feminism in the 1960s and 1970s. The associated emphasis of the civil rights and idea that the personal is political that that was present during that time in U.S. history impacted Rogers, her theory development, and the conceptualization of theories to com.

According to O'Hara (2016), "Ahead of her dad, and pretty much his teacher on this, Natalie was keenly aware of the political implications of the person-centered principles. She had an exquisitely tuned antenna for the power dynamics in a group that makes space for some voices and silences others" (p. 562). Rogers believed in the power of action in addition to intention, and she was often more confrontational and verbal about injustice than her father was. She was a social justice pioneer who truly believed in and lived the concept of the *personal as political.* Refusing to ride on the coattails of her father, Rogers chose to live creatively, authentically, and courageously. Her authenticity inspired others to release their own creativity and inner truths. O'Hara (2016) paid tribute to Rogers's contributions with this succinct encapsulation of Rogers's legacy:

> And surely now more than ever that expanded view of what it means to be a person—our feelings, rationality, embodiment, intuition, creativity and courage—must enliven and inspire a new generation as we seek to recover our humanity in a world that increasingly dehumanizes. (p. 565)

THEORIST BIOGRAPHY: LAURA PERLS

Laura Perls was born Laura Posner in summer 1905 and passed away in summer 1990 at the age of eighty-four. She was born in Pforzeim, Germany, but after meeting her husband Fritz, she fled with him from Nazi Germany to Holland. From there, the Perlses moved to South Africa where they lived for more than a decade. It was there that they began developing Gestalt theory. Eventually, the Perlses crossed the ocean to continue their work in New York City. While New York City became Laura Perls's home base, her husband continued to travel frequently and eventually settled on the West Coast of the United States (Bernard, 1986; Serlin, 1992).

Key Concepts and Utilization of Theory

While Fritz Perls wandered about the globe professing his theory, it was Laura Perls who nurtured the New York School of Gestalt Therapy, establishing this theory within the United States. According to Rosenblatt (1980), "Just as she maintained a home for her children, so she maintained a home for the fledgling Institute; indeed, for decades meetings were held in her living room" (p. 6). During the final year of her life, Perls returned to her place of origin in Pforzeim, Germany, where her daughter cared for her until her death in that small town in which she had been born. Serlin (1992) remarked that although Perls wrote less than her husband did regarding Gestalt theory, her contributions, from the conception to establishment of the theory, were significant. Furthermore, "because women's narratives are often not heard, and because Laura wrote very little, it is important to tell her story" (Serlin, 1992,

p. 57). Her story is illuminated in her writings, as well as the valuable insight she provided during interviews and in her collected works. Comparing herself to her husband, Perls commented, "I am less theatrical but more thorough in a lot of ways" (Bernard, 1986, p. 370). Where Fritz Perls left off with Gestalt theoretical constructs, Laura Perls followed through, applying the constructs in meaningful, sustainable ways.

Within the context of Gestalt theory, Laura Perls emphasized the concept of *support*. While her husband's demonstrations of Gestalt therapy often highlighted the roles of action, confrontation, and experiments in heightening awareness and provoking contact, Perls focused on the importance of having appropriate *support* during this process (Serlin, 1992). Perls stated that the therapist "should only experiment to the degree that support is available" (Bernard, 1986, p. 371). By *support*, Perls meant the therapist's role in activating the client's internal psychological support. Being a true humanist, Perls believed that clients had the internal ability to *support* themselves, physically and metaphorically, and that the therapist's job was to bring this realization about by being empathic, present, and available (Bernard, 1986; Serlin, 1992). Perls (1992) wrote,

> Support starts with primary physiology like breathing, circulation, and digestion, continues with the development of the cortex, the growing of teeth, upright posture, coordination, sensitivity and mobility, language and its uses, habits and customs, even and particularly the hang-ups which were formed as support at the time of their formation. (p. 54)

Through the processes of learning, *assimilation*, and integration, supports are built up internally throughout the lifetime.

In relation to *support,* Perls (1992) spoke of organismic *energy* and the idea that *energy* becomes blocked within clients, noting, "The task of therapy is to develop sufficient support for the reorganization and re-channeling of energy" (p. 51). The process of becoming aware of blocked *energy* is supported through *organismic self-regulation*, whereby clients become focused and aware of what it is that they need to survive. They are then able to use *energy* to make *contact* with their environments in order to *assimilate* and fulfill their needs. Perls (1992) explained *contact* as well as the concept of a *boundary* by saying, "Contact is the recognition of, and the coping with the *other*, the different, the new, the strange. It is not a state that we are in or out of, but an activity. I make contact on the boundary between me and the other. The boundary is where we touch and at the same time experience separateness" (p. 53). The boundary is where what an individual was previously unaware of comes into focus, receives the *energy* of the individual's attention, and can thus be freely and responsibly dealt with through that *awareness*.

Perls emphasized the importance of the *awareness continuum* in maintaining psychological health and easing pathology. As clients gain awareness and make contact at their boundaries, they are able to utilize the necessary supports to ease the discomfort and necessary tension that learning and experiencing entail. Perls (1992) stated, "Contact can be relevant and creative only to the extent that support for it is available" (p. 54). To this end, Perls emphasized the importance of being uncomfortable, dissonant, or *embarrassed*, as she believed that such a state of tension leads to responsive *creativity* and growth. "Embarrassment," Perls wrote, "has become for me a creative state. It is the boundary state par excellence. You are always with one foot in what you know and one foot in what you don't know. Actually, any development starts with disequilibrium. If there is complete homeostasis, nothing happens" (as cited in Serlin, 1992, p. 62). Essentially, it is *support* that eases the tension from the *energy* (positive or negative) happening at the boundary, which in turn allows the client to learn, *assimilate*, and develop healthily. Ultimately, Perls believed that to be healthy, clients must develop more *elastic support functions* that enable them to be more at ease with uncertainty. She described this as simply learning "to live with *uncertainty without anxiety*" (Perls, 1992, p. 55). Although this state may be temporarily uncomfortable, it is survivable and an essential part of the process of living and growing.

Subversive Nature of Theories

Laura Perls was subversive on multiple levels. As Bandin (2010) suggested, the Gestalt approach was subversive in that it was an alternative to psychoanalysis and the Perlses' rebelliousness became a hallmark of the Gestalt identity. As a couple, the Perlses experienced dissonance; their relationship has been characterized as troubled and polarizing (Rosanes-Berrett, 1993). Some of this contentiousness may have been due to the lack of acknowledgment of Laura Perls's contributions to Gestalt theory. According to Perls herself, "I was in on everything in the beginning, and we discussed everything together. However, I left most of what I produced to Fritz" (Bernard, 1986, p. 369). Among Laura Perls's many contributions are two chapters from Fritz Perls's first book, *Ego, Hunger, and Aggression* (1969), which Perls authored independently from her husband yet received no acknowledgment. Laura Perls was honest about her troubled marriage, noting, "For some years I felt somewhat resentful that he never acknowledged my collaboration in the whole development of Gestalt therapy" (Bernard, 1986, p. 370).

The lack of credit given to Laura Perls and women in general is illuminated in Serlin's (1992) tribute to Laura Perls:

> Laura lived a full life, yet wrote very little, and little has been written about her. This lack of written documentation by and about women figures in history has been noted by feminist critics in the field of literary criticism. These critics take up the question of why women writers write less than men or do not think that their lives are worth describing. The narrative of Laura's life, therefore, can be understood in the context of the recent effort to move the narratives of women's lives and accomplishments from background to foreground. (p. 58)

Laura Perls would have concurred with this sentiment. She stated, "I still think that if women are to achieve anything in the professions now, they must be smarter and more persistent than many men who make it, sometimes with minimal gifts" (Bernard, 1986, p. 372). Despite these challenges, Perls's strength of spirit and tenacity allowed her to remain in contact with her truths and retain her legacy, as she responded creatively to both internal and external barriers to being seen, heard, and remembered. It may be that part of Perls's creative response to allow her husband to take credit for Gestalt theory initially and claim credit for her contributions later. This may be viewed as a type of subversive strategy, perhaps, unique to Perls, and additional evidence of her creativity. Practitioners of counseling and psychotherapy are undoubtedly in her debt for her sustained efforts to establish Gestalt theory; apply the theory in a more thorough, comprehensive manner; and courageously speak her own truths.

REFERENCES

Anthony, L. (2015). Natalie Rogers. *Therapy Today*, *26*(9), 40.

Bandín, C. V. (2010). Reflections on process groups at the 11th International Gestalt Therapy Conference ("The Union of Differences"), Madrid, April 2009. *Gestalt Review*, *14*(2), 196–203. https://www.jstor.org/stable/10.5325/gestaltreview.14.2.0196

Bernard, J. M. (1986). Laura Perls: From ground to figure. *Journal of Counseling & Development*, *64*(6), 367–373. doi:10.1002/j.1556-6676.1986.tb01136.x

Merry, T. (1997). Counselling and creativity: An interview with Natalie Rogers. *British Journal of Guidance & Counselling*, *25*(2), 263–273. doi:10.1080/03069889708253807

O'Hara, M. (2016). Natalie Rogers: Artist, healer, activist, 1927–2015. *Journal of Humanistic Psychology*, *56*(5), 561–566. doi:10.1177%2F0022167816639420

Perls, L. (1992). Concepts and misconceptions of Gestalt therapy. *Journal of Humanistic Psychology*, *32*(3), 50–56. doi:10.1177%2F0022167892323004

Rogers, N., Tudor, K., Tudor, L., & Keemar, K. (2012). Person-centered expressive arts therapy: A theoretical encounter. *Person-Centered & Experiential Psychotherapies*, *11*(1), 31–47. doi:10.1080/14779757.2012.656407

Rosanes-Berrett, M. B. (1993). Reflections on Fritz Perls: A response to Laura Perls and Ilene Serlin. *Journal of Humanistic Psychology, 33*(1), 106–109. doi:10.1177/0022167893331007

Rosenblatt, D. (1980). Introduction. *The Gestalt Journal, 3*(1), 5–15.

Serlin, I. A. (1992). Tribute to Laura Perls. *Journal of Humanistic Psychology, 32*(3), 57–66. doi:10.1177/0022167892323005

Sommers-Flanagan, J. (2007). The development and evolution of person-centered expressive art therapy: A conversation with Natalie Rogers. *Journal of Counseling & Development, 85*(1), 120–125. doi:10.1002/j.1556-6678.2007.tb00454.x

Chapter 4

Cognitive Behavioral Theorists

Cognitive behavioral therapy (CBT) represents a natural progression from behavioral therapy. As scholars began to look at humanity in a more prosocial and holistic manner, behavioral techniques were mixed with cognitive and emotive techniques to create a new genre of psychotherapy interventions called cognitive behavioral therapy. CBT includes cognitive therapy and dialectical behavioral therapy. While Aaron Beck is credited as the father of cognitive therapy, it is his daughter, Judith S. Beck (1954–present), who advanced his mission by serving as president of the Beck Institute for Cognitive Behavior Therapy and publishing works that address using CBT techniques in areas such as personality disorders and weight loss. Marsha Linehan (1943–present) developed dialectical behavioral therapy which is a psychotherapy technique that helps clients to regulate their emotions and decrease conflict in relationships. Dialectical behavioral therapy is well researched and considered a top modality in working with individuals with personality disorders such as borderline personality disorder, as well as diagnoses such as depression, post-traumatic stress disorder, and eating disorders. Linehan combined mindfulness practice with behavioral and cognitive techniques in order to create dialectical behavioral therapy. While there have been many women associated with the utilization of and advancement of cognitive and behavioral techniques, there are two women who have contributed to the theoretical foundations of these techniques: Judith S. Beck and Marsha Linehan.

THEORIST BIOGRAPHY: JUDITH S. BECK

Judith S. Beck was born in 1954 in Philadelphia, Pennsylvania. Her father Aaron is the founder of cognitive therapy (CT). Limited information is available on her mother, childhood, family, children, and personal life.

Key Concepts and Utilization of Theory

Judith is best known for her development of CT into a modern therapeutic modality. Beck is the current president of the nonprofit Beck Institute for Cognitive Behavior Therapy. Beck began her career as a teacher for children with learning disabilities. After earning a master's degree and doctorate in psychology, Beck opened the Beck Institute for Cognitive Behavior Therapy with her father in 1994. She is the institute's president and travels the world teaching practitioners about CT and its uses.

Beck has described CBT as collaborative, structured, goal-oriented, and as short term as possible. One of the main components of CBT involves challenging automatic thoughts. Counseling sessions follow a specific format. According to Beck, "[Clinicians] ask about the patient's mood; make a bridge between sessions; set a specific problem-solving-oriented agenda; work toward solving specific problems; collaboratively set homework assignments (so patients can make small changes in their thinking and behavior every day); and summarize and ask for feedback at the end of sessions" (as cited in Sussman, 2006). Beck also outlined the specific progression of sessions as outlined in table 4.1.

Table 4.1 Progression of Cognitive Behavioral Sessions

First session	Establish rapport, educate client about any diagnoses they have been given, explain cognitive behavioral theory, obtain client goals for treatment, and instill hope.
Following sessions:	Compare client's current state versus that of previous sessions (using both interviewing and tests such as the Beck Depression Inventory) and perform a symptom check.
Next:	Set an agenda with client and discuss any other impacting issues Review week between sessions. Discuss completed homework.
Finally:	Rank agenda items and begin discussing them based on importance. Based on the problem at hand, teach the client cognitive and behavioral skills. Collaboratively assign homework. At the end of the session, review helpful moments from the session with the client and ask for client feedback about the session and the counselor's actions.

Theoretical Constructs

The main construct of CBT is that thoughts, feelings, and behaviors are interconnected and in order to heal, a client must recognize and rework feelings that lead to automatic thoughts. In this way, the client's behaviors become consistent with the client's wishes. This goal-oriented theory allows the counselor and the client to almost immediately tackle the problem at hand and to identify new ways of reacting to and thinking about the issue. Clinicians often take a teaching role, and clients are often given homework to complete between sessions.

Subversive Nature of Theory

While Aaron Beck is famous for developing CBT, it is Judith Beck who has worked to bring the theory into a more public domain. She has published many books on the topic of weight loss and CBT and has dedicated her career to ensuring proper training for clinicians who are utilizing her theory.

THEORIST BIOGRAPHY: MARSHA LINEHAN

Marsha Linehan was born in 1943 in Tulsa, Oklahoma. She is best known for creating dialectical behavior therapy (DBT). At the age seventeen, Linehan was admitted to inpatient care at the Institute of Living in Hartford, Connecticut, due to self-harm and extreme social withdrawal. She stated she was incorrectly diagnosed with schizophrenia; she believed a more accurate diagnosis would have been borderline personality disorder. She received her undergraduate degree, master's degree, and doctoral degrees at Loyola University Chicago. Employed by various universities in the United States, she focused her research on borderline personality disorder and individuals with severe suicidal ideation. Her own diagnosis coupled with her psychological education background led her to the creation of DBT.

Key Concepts and Utilization of Theory

Linehan was praying in a church in Chicago when she was struck with a new sense of self-compassion. Reflecting on how she progressed from her teenage years to that moment, she hypothesized that the biggest influence on her mental health had been her radical self-acceptance. This moment spawned the creation of her theory called DBT. As her theory solidified, she began utilizing it with clients who were experiencing severe suicidal ideation and found that DBT decreased suicidal tendencies more effectively than other forms of psychotherapy. Linehan stated,

> I decided to get supersuicidal people, the very worst cases, because I figured these are the most miserable people in the world. They think they're evil, that they're bad, bad, bad and I understood that they weren't. I understood their suffering because I'd been there, in hell, with no idea how to get out. (Carey, 2011, para. 35)

DBT is a cognitive behavioral treatment that includes "individual psychotherapy, group skills training, telephone coaching, and a therapist consultation team" (Linehan, 2014, p. 3). The name comes from the word "dialectics," meaning both the nature of reality and dialogue within relationships. Dialectics makes three basic assumptions: "All things are interconnected, change is constant and inevitable, and opposites can be integrated to form a closer approximation of the truth" (Schimelpfening, 2019, para. 5). DBT is well researched and has been found to be efficacious in treating issues such as mood disorders, borderline personality disorder, suicidality, and substance abuse.

DBT's main goals are the development of mindfulness, interpersonal effectiveness, emotion regulation, and distress tolerance skills. These skills can be taught to a client using a specific program outlined in texts such as Linehan's *DBT Skills Training Manual* (2014). A core concept of DBT is radical acceptance: the clinician's profound acknowledgement of the client and the client's revolutionary recognition of themself. Linehan explained radical acceptance by stating, "Suppressing what you want is not the way to go. You have to radically accept that you want something you don't have and that it's not a catastrophe" (Linehan, 2017, p. 243). She believed that it is not necessary for an individual to stop trying to change things, but the individual does have to accept a moment and then work toward change as part of this life-changing construct.

Subversive Nature of Theory

DBT is a modality of psychotherapy and counseling that is often used with diagnoses that are mistakenly thought to be "women's issues," such as borderline personality disorder and eating disorders. The reality, of course, is although more women than men are given these diagnoses, this may be because of client underreporting, clinician bias, and gendered societal expectations. Additionally, DBT's focus on spirituality and intimate communication can be a deterrent for people who are impacted by the hegemonic belief that self-care and vulnerability are gendered rather than universal experiences. When Linehan chose to reveal her own experience with borderline personality disorder, she instantly put the lie to the claim that in order to be a helper, an individual must be issue-free (an idea that while false, is nevertheless prevalent). Her act of vulnerability highlights the core of her theory: One must radically accept themselves in order to begin the process of changing and healing.

Linehan's choice to reveal this personal information about herself was unique. Personal disclosure on the part of a clinician, particularly as it relates to mental health, was strongly discouraged. There was a clear distinction between personal and professional. The position of the professional clinician, particularly with cognitive therapies, was a powerful knowing person who would be in the position of expert in the therapeutic relationship. The stigma associated with mental health issues was the dominant discourse at the time and disclosing a mental health diagnosis would be considered a weakness, thus demonstrating the radical nature of Linehan's radical acceptance found within her theory.

It is interesting to note that there are similarities between Beck and Linehan aside from both currently contributing and impacting CT as a whole. Both Beck and Linehan focus on reaching as many people as they can, but in very different ways. In Beck's case, this is through workshops and new applications. In Linehan's case this is through personal vulnerability. Through reaching so many others, Beck and Linehan continue to expand and promote their theories within counseling and psychotherapy.

REFERENCES

Beck, J. S. (2011). Cognitive-behavioral therapy. *Clinical Textbook of Addictive Disorders*, 491, 474–501.

Carey, B. (2011). Expert on mental illness reveals her own fight. *The New York Times*. https://www.nytimes.com/2011/06/23/health/23lives.html

Dimeff, L., & Linehan, M. M. (2001). Dialectical behavior therapy in a nutshell. *The California Psychologist*, *34*(3), 10–13. https://www.researchgate.net/profile/Marsha_Linehan/publication/239279018_Dialectical_Behavior_Therapy_in_a_Nutshell/links/00463530be15f63c28000000.pdf

Dimeff, L. A., & Koerner, K. E. (2007). *Dialectical Behavior Therapy in Clinical Practice: Applications Across Disorders and Settings*. Guilford Press.

Graham, J. R., Sorenson, S., & Hayes-Skelton, S. A. (2013). Enhancing the cultural sensitivity of cognitive behavioral interventions for anxiety in diverse populations. *The Behavior Therapist/AABT*, *36*(5), 101–108. https://www.ncbi.nlm.nih.gov/pmc/articles/PMC4225557/

Linehan, M. (2014). *DBT Skills Training Manual*. Guilford Publications.

Linehan, M. (2017). Marsha Linehan: How she learned radical acceptance [Video file]. *BorderlinerNotes*. https://youtu.be/OTG7YEWkJFI

Madewell, J., & Shaughnessy, M. F. (2009). An interview with Judith Beck about cognitive therapy: Judith Beck. *North American Journal of Psychology*, *11*(1), 29–36.

Schimelpfening, N. (2019). What to know about dialectical behavior therapy. *Verywell Mind.* https://www.verywellmind.com/dialectical-behavior-therapy-1067402

Sussman, N. (2006). In session with Judith S. Beck, PhD: Cognitive-behavioral therapy. *Primary Psychiatry, 13(4)*, 31–34.

Telch, C. F., Agras, W. S., & Linehan, M. M. (2001). Dialectical behavior therapy for binge eating disorder. *Journal of Consulting and Clinical Psychology, 69*(6), 1061–1065. doi:10.1037/0022-006X.69.6.1061

Chapter 5

Postmodern Theorists

Postmodernism questioned many of the historical, philosophical, and epistemological premises and Western contexts of counseling theories. Postmodernism supports multiple perspectives and encourages discursive analysis of the influence of language, culture, and power. Postmodern models are grounded in the idea that knowledge and meaning are constructed through interactions with others. A leading goal of postmodern theories is to give power back to clients, allowing them to voice their own stories. Two of the theories developed in the postmodern era are solution-focused brief therapy and narrative therapy. This chapter seeks to amplify the voices of two women clinicians and theorists, Insoo Kim Berg and Cheryl White. Insoo Kim Berg (1934–2007) was a Korean-born American psychotherapist, lecturer, and author. She was married to Steve de Shazer and was a key innovator in the development of SFBT. She and de Shazer co-founded the Brief Family Therapy Center in Milwaukee, Wisconsin. Across the globe, Cheryl White was married to Michael White, a leading figure in the development of narrative therapy. White and her husband met while both were pursuing degrees in social work. They co-founded the Dulwich Centre in Adelaide, Australia. White was with him when narrative therapy was developed. She founded Dulwich Centre Publications in 1984, a publisher that specializes in works that challenge dominant cultural understandings and represent a diversity of cultures and sexual and gender orientations. Dulwich Centre Publications seeks to document the history of narrative therapy and of therapeutic and community work ideas and practices in ways that assist practitioners.

THEORIST BIOGRAPHY: INSOO KIM BERG

Insoo Kim Berg (née Kim) was born on July 25, 1934, in Seoul, Korea. She passed away on January 10, 2007, in Wauwatosa, Wisconsin, at the age of seventy-two. Berg was born into an affluent Korean Presbyterian family that strongly valued education. Her family was in the pharmaceutical manufacturing business, and Berg was selected to be the family pharmacist. She was interested in and excelled in chemistry and was a pharmacy major at Ewha Woman's University in Seoul. In 1957, she came to the United States to continue her pharmacy studies. Soon after her arrival, she married her first husband, Charles H. Berg, and gave birth to her daughter Sarah. Berg was raised to believe that everyone's parents decided what their children were going to study and that children obeyed their parents' wishes. After she came to the United States, she was shocked to discover that students were able to decide this for themselves. It dawned on Berg that her parents were 6,500 miles away and had no idea what she was doing, so she switched her focus to social work. Berg did not tell her parents for a couple of years. Once they were told, although they did not understand the concept of social work, Berg's parents did not create any difficulties for Berg because Berg avoided discussing it. The way she addressed this issue in her family exemplifies a core belief of solution-focused brief therapy (SFBT), which is to avoid focusing on problems.

Key Concepts and Utilization of Theory

Berg was described by her good friend Yvonne Dolan as "a tiny Korean woman with short dark hair, twinkling eyes and a gentle, caring manner" (Durrant, 2007, p. 3). She was further characterized as an enthusiastic, optimistic, and tenacious woman who never seemed to stop working. Other personal characteristics included a tirelessly positive attitude and a deep respect for the competence, resourcefulness, and self-knowledge found within every person. Berg earned her bachelor of science and master of social work degrees from the University of Wisconsin, Milwaukee, and completed postgraduate studies at the Family Institute of Chicago, the Menninger Foundation in Kansas, and the Mental Research Institute (MRI) in California, where she was supervised by John Weakland. It was at MRI that Berg learned about the development of brief therapy approaches and met her second husband, Steve de Shazer. She and de Shazer moved back to Milwaukee, de Shazer's hometown, and with their colleagues, they co-founded the Brief Family Therapy Center (BFTC). Berg contributed to SFBT by drawing on her Korean heritage, scientific mind, and direct communication skills. She was active in marriage and family therapy and authored many articles and books. Berg traveled often and conducted seminars and workshops on SFBT throughout Asia, Canada, Europe, South America, and the United States.

As its name implies, SFBT is a short-term approach and one that does not seek to uncover problems or unresolved issues in individuals or families. A foundational concept of SFBT is that the client sets the goals in therapy and those goals determine the course of the therapy. The underlying assumptions of SFBT are that each client is the expert on their own life, there is no one right way to live, and the therapist is not the expert and does not have an agenda or make judgments about the client's goals. Berg believed that clients have all the components of a solution within them but do not have the necessary awareness. She believed that through SFBT, a client could learn to see each of the components and develop their own pathway for reaching a solution. If a solution does not work, the client is encouraged to do something different. When a client has identified a solution that works, the therapist encourages the client to do more of that.

SFBT focuses on solutions and not problems. This singular focus was developed from Berg's experiences working in community mental health, substance dependency programs, homeless and domestic shelters, correction departments, and family service programs. Berg enjoyed and felt comfortable working with clients in these environments. Most of the clients had many challenges and faced many issues, and they had neither the interest nor the resources to spend time helping a therapist fully understand their problems. It is understandable, then, that instead of adding to a client's issues by thinking about problems, she focused on helping the client to build their own solutions. A unique concept in SFBT is that there is no connection between a problem and the solution. Berg believed that regardless of the particulars of a client's problem, the solution necessarily included individuals talking to each other and getting along (Yalom & Rubin, 2003). However, Berg discovered the paths individuals take to reach solutions vary greatly.

The miracle question. The SFBT approach encourages therapists to describe what life might look like without the problems that their clients have identified. It is through this concept that Berg invented the miracle question. Although this intervention has been adapted and applied in many situations, her original miracle question is as follows:

> Suppose a miracle happens overnight, tonight when you go to bed. And all the problems that brought you here to talk to me today are gone. Disappeared. But because this happens while you were sleeping, you have no idea that there was a miracle during the night. The problem is all gone, all solved. See when you are slowly waking up, coming out of your sleep, what might be the first, small clue that will make you think, "Oh my gosh. There must have been a miracle during the night. The problem is all gone!" (Yalom & Rubin, 2003)

A client shares descriptions of how they would know that their problems were gone, and the therapist encourages the development of the client's story with questions that expand the social context. For instance, the therapist might ask how the client's family (e.g., colleagues, neighbors, community members) would come to know that the client had experienced a miracle during the night. Using this SFBT intervention, the client can begin to visualize how to reach a better place. The therapist concludes with the question to the client about what they need to do to get this started.

Unlike many other theories, SFBT does not place an emphasis on the therapeutic relationship as an instrument of change. Berg did not believe in the strength of the therapist-client relationship because rather than being a lifelong bond, the relationship is as short as possible. She thought that rather than clients spending time talking to their therapists about why they do not have friends, they need to live their lives and begin trying to make friendships work. Berg described the process of change as being "as minimalistic as possible"; she was "not interested in overhauling personality. . . . Most people just have a little quirk here or there that doesn't work" (Yalom & Rubin, 2003). There is an underlying assumption in SFBT that individuals want to have better lives. The role of the therapist is to help the client down a path that facilitates this. SFBT does not focus on obstacles to change; rather, the SFBT therapist helps the client find goals that are very small and realistic. One way to accomplish this is through exception questions.

Just as the name implies, exception questions are used by SFBT therapists to encourage clients to describe their experiences with exceptions to their problems or solutions that have worked, even if they only worked one time. The focus is on gathering details and information regarding successful resolutions to the client's problem and the context. By reminding the client that there was a time when the problem did not impact them as much or was not present, the therapist instills hope. The exception questions can also help a client recall specific details that are useful for finding ideas and components with which to build a current solution or plan.

Berg did not present SFBT as an approach that works for everyone. A criticism of SFBT is that if a therapist does not spend time listening to a client's problems or stories about the past, the client may not feel heard, understood, or ready for change. In this case, the therapist has not met the client where they are. However, Berg believed that when a client makes an appointment, they realize that what they are doing currently is not working, have decided to make a change, and hope to find a solution. Many problems are grounded in culture, and postmodern theories generally examine how society exerts power over some marginalized groups within a particular context. The SFBT premise that the client is the expert gives the client power, which in turn facilitates safety. SFBT is social justice–oriented in that the client is able to voice their ideas.

Berg taught SFBT in many countries, and she believed that SFBT needed only minor modifications to address the cultural differences among these countries. Consistent with SFBT's focus on solutions rather than problems, Berg focused on similarities between cultures and peoples rather than differences. She preferred focusing on humans' shared basic needs, goals, and aspirations, such as acceptance, validation, support, love, and belongingness. Berg provided examples of individual differences with a single cultural group (e.g., every Korean family is not the same) just as often as she did variations between groups. She viewed each person as a unique human being rather than a part of a group. Berg found focusing on differences very divisive and said, "I don't pay attention to that" (Yalom & Rubin, 2003).

Subversive Nature of Theory

Berg was trained in psychoanalysis and taught to focus on individuals' problems, which was the usual psychotherapy practice at that time. Her family therapy theory evolved from her individual therapy practice, but she maintained psychoanalytic concepts such as a person's undifferentiated ego mass. Berg experienced many failures using a psychoanalytic approach, and as an extremely bright academic who had known only success her whole life, failure was not part of her narrative or self-concept. Through her failures, she came to see that most of her clients were not in a place to be engaging in introspection, nor were they interested in developing insights or engaging in personal growth. Berg discovered that it does not help for a therapist to talk to a person about what is wrong with them, as Berg herself been trained; the client just wants the problem to go away. Berg's past success in handling her own family problems coupled with her experiences using the family theories of the day led her to strive to do something different.

Similar to how Linehan discussed in chapter 4 on cognitive behavioral theorists, used her own experiences to inform the development of Dialectical Behavioral Therapy, Berg used her own experiences to inform her theoretical conceptualizations. In drawing on her personal experience in the creation of SFBT, Berg was bucking the scientific zeitgeist of the times that prioritized objectivity above all else. Berg went directly against current therapies focused on problems to instead focus on solutions. She actively changed her techniques to develop her own therapeutic style. Berg was referred to by de Shazer as gifted clinician; he said that he learned how to do therapy from watching Berg work. Toward the end of his life, de Shazer shared that he had spent his thirty-year career trying to accurately identify Berg's clinical skills and interventions so that others might learn how she did SFBT (Dolan, 2007). However, when SFBT is discussed in theory textbooks, de Shazer is presented first and receives the bulk of the credit. Berg is presented second and is usually initially referred to as his wife and only then as a SFBT clinician. It is likely that this presentation is due to the gender roles and social norms of Berg and de Shazer's time. Women were just beginning to work outside of the home and have their own careers, and Berg worked with her husband. It appears in retrospect that SFBT's original concepts and ideas were developed by Berg and that these concepts and ideas were documented and presented to the world by de Shazer. In a tribute to Berg after her death, one of Berg's close colleagues, Michael Durrant, said that SFBT revolutionized the therapy world and that this was Berg's mission and "her miracle" (Durant, 2007, p. 3).

The ideas Berg presented were considered radical; indeed, she described herself as way out on the left side. The idea of focusing on the positive, conducting only one or two therapy sessions, avoiding exploring the past or the unconscious ego, and giving unique homework assignments were considered very unconventional in light of the psychodynamic and family theories prevalent at that time. Other professionals were threatened by Berg and did not take her seriously, which contributed to her self-doubt. Decades later during an interview, Berg reminisced about how she was trained to focus on what was wrong with individuals. While this was the therapeutic norm of her peers, Berg rejected it, stating, "No, I don't want to join that pack."

THEORIST BIOGRAPHY: CHERYL WHITE

Cheryl White was born and raised in Australia in the 1950s. Her birth name and birthdate are not publicly available, and little has been written about her. What is known is that White was part of the first generation in her family to complete high school or to have any formal college education (White, 2016a). White attended the University of Australia where she pursued a degree in social work. While there, she met Michael White. She and Michael married, and in 1983 they established the Dulwich Centre in Adelaide as a base for pursuing their interests in psychotherapy and community work.

Key Concepts and Utilization of Theory

In 1984, Cheryl White founded Dulwich Centre Publications (DCP) as an independent, feminist-owned publishing company. The Whites worked together and collaborated with others for more than two decades on the development of narrative therapy (NT). The Whites separated in 2007, and Michael White passed away early in 2008. Cheryl White continued the work of NT, serving as director of the Dulwich Centre and the secretary of the

Dulwich Centre Foundation, finding applications of narrative therapy with diverse groups and communities. She continues to work as a publisher, editor, teacher, training coordinator, conference host, and initiator of projects at DCP (Dulwich Centre, n.d.). She is the author and co-editor of several books and publisher of many more.

The NT approach focuses on the stories people tell themselves and others about their lives. As a postmodern theory, NT is grounded in the concept that reality is socially constructed through individuals' interactions and dialogue with others. What may be true for one person may not be true for another person, and a core belief of NT is that all perspectives and truths are valid. Individuals may create narrowly focused problem-saturated stories about events in their lives, and in turn may internalize these stories such that they become their identity and self-narrative. NT seeks to separate or externalize the problem from the person; deconstruct the story; understand the social, cultural, and political contexts; and empower the person to develop or reauthor an alternative new story (White & Epston, 1990).

NT therapists respect clients and believe they are competent and capable experts on their own lives. It is normal to experience problems, so no fault or blame is placed on clients or anyone else. However, individuals may simplify and personalize events without an awareness of the broader complex contexts that influence situations. Considering the dominant cultural discourses that relate to problems provides a different perspective and leads clients to a deeper and thicker understanding that is less personal. The overlays of historical, social, and political influences are deconstructed and examined as contextual and contributing factors to client problems. The client leads the therapeutic sessions, and the NT therapist focuses on the client's story and the effects of the problem rather than the causes, playing the role of a collaborative listener and investigative reporter. NT therapists ask questions to facilitate the client process of uncovering values and strengths. They seek exceptions to problem-saturated interpretations and unique outcomes of instances in which clients are able to overcome their problems (Perjessy, 2017; White & Epston, 1990).

NT positions a therapist to listen to the stories of their clients within the clients' cultural contexts. NT is especially well-suited to cultures in which individuals experience problems due to socially constructed hierarchies such as racism and sexism. Individuals can give voice to their stories as their truths, externalize negative cultural messages as their problems, and gain awareness of the power of cultural systems in their lives. The goal of therapy is for a client to develop multiple storylines and ultimately reauthor their story (Semmler & Williams, 2000; White & Epston, 1990). It is in this focus on gender and cultural contexts that Cheryl White's influence becomes evident.

Subversive Nature of Theory

It may be inconsistent with NT to use the word "subversive" to describe this subsection due to NT's sensitivity to language and respectful and blame-free approach to individuals. However, as White (2016b) wrote in her letter to the readers of the memory book for narrative practice, "Any field of practice also involves multiple histories" (p. 8). It would thus be consistent with NT to validate all stories and perspectives, to provide historical and cultural contexts, and to develop an alternative story that thickens and enriches the narrative. White places emphasis on gender and culture, inviting women of many cultures to share their stories of hope and complexity, yet these contributions have remained relatively out of focus in textbooks and teachings on NT in graduate education. This subsection provides another version of history that relies on intentionally listening to White's voice and attending to her contributions to NT.

Cheryl White was Michael White's personal and professional partner; therefore, it is conceivable that her contributions to NT are embedded in the presentation of her husband's ideas. As with many partnerships and relationships, it can be difficult to know where one partner ends and the other begins. White and her husband's unique voices may be so interwoven in the discourse of NT that it is impossible to separate them. White was present when it all began in 1980, engaging in dialogue and processing ideas with her husband and Ann and David Epston every step of the way in the development of NT.

While her husband was extroverted and appeared to be energized by speaking to large audiences, White herself was relational and quiet, engaging in deeper conversations and making stronger connections with individuals and small groups. In their work on NT, the couple traveled the world and met with diverse cultural and theoretical leaders. It was in these spaces of dialogue that White gained insight into the social and political contexts of issues that inform individuals' narratives and stories. White's attention to gender and culture is evident in the incorporation of these concepts into NT.

Being a woman allowed White to influenced NT and engage with feminist issues during the theory's development. She experienced the feminist movement of the 1970s and 1980s, which attended to the problems of gender roles, gender inequities, and gendered language. She experienced these issues personally and placed them into the broader social and political contexts of oppression. White became aware of the societal norms that conveyed to women that they were not in charge of their own bodies. Gaining knowledge about issues such as contraceptive use, abortion, sexual decision-making, and birth options affected White profoundly. It is difficult to imagine that NT would have embraced discourse related to language and gender had White not influenced her husband's ideas.

White has acknowledged the contributions of many individuals from a variety of cultures to the field of narrative practice, referring to the field of narrative practice as a tapestry (White, 2016b). Some of the threads are from White's dialogue with Paulo Freire. Freire was a Brazilian educator who was known for his advocacy of critical pedagogy. White was present at his last interview. She reflected on Freire's charge to look for answers in the right places and began to question how individuals might be able to respond to stories of social suffering in ways that not only alleviate their own sorrow but also address in some way broader injustices, violence, and abuses. Other threads of NT stem from White's relationship with America Bracho, a Venezuelan medical doctor who is reshaping culturally appropriate physical health services by transferring power and responsibility for healthcare to laypeople via the dissemination of information. White's lessons from Freire and Bracho have helped shape NT's attention to the social constructs that influence the contexts of problem-saturated stories and the transfer of power from the therapist to the client, who is the expert on their own life. It has been more than a decade since her husband's death, and White continues to seek out diverse voices and a robust community in the hope of further innovations, creativities, and generative partnerships. She is particularly interested in finding ways to support the work of practitioners in difficult contexts (Dulwich Centre, n.d.; White, 2016b).

White is the first to acknowledge the many other contributors to the development of NT. She has spent most of her career privileging voices other than her own. This subsection is but a brief glimpse into how White has influenced the direction and the development of NT.

The two women covered in this chapter, Berg and White, contributed to postmodern theory development. A similarity they have in common is that both Berg and White avoid focusing on the problem that the client presents. Moving away from the surface problem or behavioral issue represents a departure from previous types of counseling and psychotherapy. How these two theorists differ, however, is that Berg faced resistance and adversity in an overt verbal manner. In contrast, White appears to continue to quietly continue to work through publications.

REFERENCES

Berg, I. K. (1994). *Family-Based Services: A Solution-Focused Approach*. Norton.

Berg, I. K., & de Jong, P. (1996). Solution-building conversations: Co-constructing a sense of competence with clients. *Families in Society*, *77*(6), 376–391. doi:10.1606/1044-3894.934

Berg, I. K., & de Shazer, S. (1993). Making numbers talk: Language in therapy. In S. Friedman (ed.), *The New Language of Change: Constructive Collaboration in Psychotherapy* (pp. 5–24). Guilford Press.

Berg, I. K., & Dolan, Y. (2001). *Tales of Solutions: A Collection of Hope-Inspiring Stories*. Norton.

Berg, I. K., & Kelly, S. (2000). *Building Solutions in Child Protective Services*. Norton.

Berg, I. K., & Miller, S. D. (1992). *Working with the Problem Drinker: A Solution-Focused Approach*. Norton.

Berg, I. K., & Reuss, N. H. (1998). *Solutions Step by Step: A Substance Abuse Treatment Manual*. Norton.

Berg, I. K., & Steiner, T. (2003). *Children's Solution Work*. Norton.

Berg, I. K., & Szabo, P. (2005). *Brief Coaching for Lasting Solutions*. Norton.

de Jong, P., & Berg, I. K. (2013). *Interviewing for Solutions* (4th edition). Brooks/Cole.

de Shazer, S., & Berg, I. K. (1995). The brief therapy tradition. In J. H. Weakland and W. A. Ray (eds.), *Propagations: Thirty Years of Influence from the Mental Research Institute* (pp. 249–252). Haworth Press.

de Shazer, S., & Berg, I. K. (1997). "What works?" Remarks on research aspects of solution-focused brief therapy. *Journal of Family Therapy*, *19*(2), 121–124. http://www.solutions-centre.org/pdf/1467-6427.00043.pdf

de Shazer, S., Berg, I. K., Lipchik, E. V. E., Nunnally, E., Molnar, A., Gingerich, W., & Weiner-Davis, M. (1986). Brief therapy: Focused solution development. *Family Process*, *25*(2), 207–221. doi:10.1111/j.1545-5300.1986.00207.x

de Shazer, S., Dolan, Y., Korman, H., McCollum, E., Trepper, T., & Berg, I. K. (2007). *More than Miracles: The State of the Art of Solution-Focused Brief Therapy*. Routledge/Haworth Press.

Dolan, Y. (2007). Tribute to Insoo Kim Berg. *Journal of Marital and Family Therapy*, *33*(2), 129. doi:10.1111/j.1752-0606.2007.00011.x

Dulwich Centre (n.d.). Our people. *Dulwich Centre*. https://dulwichcentre.com.au/about/our-people/

Durrant, M. (2007). Remembering Insoo Kim Berg. *Journal of Systemic Therapies*, *26*(2), 1–12. doi:10.1521/jsyt.2007.26.2.1

Jordan, S. S. (2017). Solution-focused brief therapy. In J. Carlson & S. B. Dermer (eds.), *The SAGE Encyclopedia of Marriage, Family, and Couples Counseling* (pp. 1575–1579). Sage Publications, Inc.

Miller, S. D., & Berg, I. K. (1996). *The Miracle Method: A Radically New Approach to Problem Drinking*. Norton.

Perjessy, C. (2017). Narrative therapy. In J. Carlson & S. B. Dermer (eds.), *The SAGE Encyclopedia of Marriage, Family, and Couples Counseling* (pp. 1133–1137). Sage Publications, Inc.

Quick, E. K. (2012). *Core Competencies in the Solution-Focused and Strategic Therapies: Becoming a Highly Competent Solution-Focused and Strategic Therapist*. Routledge.

Semmler, P. L., & Williams, C. B. (2000). Narrative therapy: A storied context for multicultural counseling. *Journal of Multicultural Counseling and Development*, *28*(1), 51–62. doi:10.1002/j.2161-1912.2000.tb00227.x

White, C. (2016a). A letter to the reader. In C. White (ed.), *A Memory Book for the Field of Narrative Practice* (pp. 6–8). Dulwich Centre Pty Limited.

White, C. (2016b). Feminist challenge and women's liberation. In C. White (ed.), *A Memory Book for the Field of Narrative Practice* (pp. 47–65). Dulwich Centre Pty Limited.

White, C., & Denborough, D. (1998). *Introducing Narrative Therapy: A Collection of Practice-Based Writings*. Dulwich Centre Publications.

White, C., & Denborough, D. (2002). *A Community of Ideas: Behind the Scenes*. Dulwich Centre Publications.

White, M., & Epston, D. (1990). *Narrative Means to Therapeutic Ends*. Norton.

Yalom, V., & Rubin, B. (2003). An interview with Insoo Kim Berg, LCSW. *Psychotherapy.net*. https://www.psychotherapy.net/interview/insoo-kim-berg

Chapter 6

Feminist and Multicultural Theorists

The end of the nineteenth century marked the beginning of modern-day psychology, with psychoanalysis established by Sigmund Freud. The development of this theory was initially informed by traditional masculine characteristics and occurred within the context of European values. It is not surprising, then, that women would not be well represented in psychological theories. Jean Baker Miller (1927–2006) was a psychiatrist who wrote about this and the social and political forces that create and influence the contexts in which ideas are developed. Miller focused on women's strengths and emphasis on relationships, infusing psychology with feminism to provide the foundation for relational-cultural theory. Miller believed that modern culture would benefit from considering the natural relational characteristics of women rather than focusing solely on clinical neutrality because healthy relationships are a human need and isolation creates psychological issues. Likewise, human behavior occurs within the framework of a culture, and multiculturalism posits that psychological problems come from society, not from within an individual. Kimberlé Crenshaw (1959–present) is an American lawyer, civil rights advocate, and leading scholar of critical race theory. Critical race theory is a framework that examines society and culture as they relate to categorizations of race, law, and power. Crenshaw coined the term "intersectionality" to explain the overlapping layers of oppression of gender and race. Her position is that Black women's experiences of race and gender cannot be understood independently of each other but must instead take into account aspects of recursive interactions between marginalized characteristics. The significant contributions of Miller and Crenshaw have expanded the influence of gender and culture on the concepts and tenets of counseling and psychotherapy theories.

THEORIST BIOGRAPHY: JEAN BAKER MILLER

Jean Baker Miller (née Baker) was born on September 29, 1927, in the Bronx, New York. She passed away on July 29, 2006, in Brookline, Massachusetts, at the age of seventy-eight. The youngest of three children, Miller was raised in a Jewish working-class family that experienced financial challenges during Miller's life. Miller was diagnosed with polio several months after her birth and spent many of her formative years in hospitals enduring painful surgeries. Miller's passion for medicine was inspired by two nurses who cared for her during that time. Miller was also inspired by many other women, including an aunt and a cousin whom she recalled as making lives for themselves outside of the home. Miller graduated from Sarah Lawrence College in 1948 and from Columbia University in 1952 with her medical degree. She completed an internship at Montefiore Hospital; residencies in medicine and psychiatry at Bellevue Medical Center, Albert Einstein College of Medicine, and Upstate Medical Center; and psychoanalytic training at the New York Medical College.

She married Mike Miller in her twenties. Mike Miller was a sociology professor who was deeply invested in poverty and inequality issues (Jordan, 2017). Together they had two sons, Jonathan and Edward. Miller had an experience while pregnant with their first son that was an indication of the role of women at the time. She was just months away from completing her training in psychiatry at Albert Einstein College of Medicine when she was asked to leave on account of her pregnancy. Miller was asked to leave singularly because of her gender and the societal views of what women who are pregnant should and should not do, even when Miller was exceeding all criteria for success in her medical training program. This unjust treatment impacted Miller and the development of her theory that highlights how characteristics of women are not valued in a culture that emphasizes the characteristics attributed to men.

Key Concepts and Utilization of Theory

After completing her education, Miller became a faculty member at Harvard Medical School and was appointed as a clinical professor of psychiatry at Boston University School of Medicine. Miller was interested in feminist ideas, and she explored psychology's failure to incorporate women's experiences. Miller edited *Psychoanalysis and Women: Contributions to New Theory and Therapy* (1973) and *Psychoanalysis and Women* (1974). In 1976, Miller authored her first book, *Toward a New Psychology of Women*, that challenged the status quo by highlighting the importance of power dynamics in human relationships. She highlighted the impact of gender and in particular, how Western culture values men's strengths but views women's strengths as weaknesses. Miller's book provided the initial ideas for a psychological theory centered on relationships and attending to cultural contexts. Miller further developed her ideas by collaborating with scholars Judith V. Jordan, Irene Stiver, and Janet Surrey in an effort to accurately represent women's experiences in mainstream psychological theories. The group was initially called the Stone Center Theory Group. It is now known as the Founding Scholars, and it is located at Wellesley College in Wellesley, Massachusetts. The group's collaborative efforts resulted in the formation of relational-cultural theory (RCT). In 1981, Miller was appointed the first director of the Stone Center of Wellesley College, where her legacy project, the Jean Baker Miller Training Institute (JBMTI), and RCT live on (JBMTI, 2019).

Miller received numerous awards during her career, including the Association for Women in Psychology Distinguished Career Award (1980), a Rockefeller Foundation fellowship (1981), the Woman of the Year Award (1982), and the American Orthopsychiatry Association Blanche F. Ittelson Memorial Award (1995). Miller wrote a second edition of *Towards a New Psychology of Women* (1987) which has since become a bestseller, translated into twenty languages, and published in twelve countries. Miller authored and coauthored numerous other works. A collection of her manuscripts can be found at the Stone Center. Miller is described as an American psychiatrist, scholar, professor, author, feminist, visionary, and social activist.

Miller's relational theory concepts were developed in response to Sigmund Freud's characterization of women as less capable than men. As a competent woman and physician, Miller opposed this characterization and others made by male contemporaries such as Sigmund Freud, Erik Erikson, and Lawrence Kohlberg, which suggested that individuals must find themselves before achieving happiness (Zeedyk & Greenwood, 2008). Miller believed women achieve happiness through their connections with others. She believed women have natural characteristics that the world needs but that women have not been encouraged to see their relationship skills as strengths. Miller challenged the hyper-individualist messages of separation and isolation prevalent in Western culture (Hartling, 2008; JMBTI, 2019; Jordan, 2017).

Miller recognized that growth-fostering connections and mutuality are important factors in psychological health and well-being. Growth-fostering connections are those supportive relationships that impact a person's life. Miller experienced this herself, believing that many of her own successes were due in part to supportive relationships. She believed growth-fostering relationships help to promote resilience, confidence, and the skills necessary to navigate new opportunities, as well as to facilitate psychological and intellectual development (Hartling, 2008). Miller identified "The Five Good Things" that characterize healthy relationships: (1) zest for those in the relationship, (2) clarity of oneself, (3) sense of worth for all in the relationship, (4) productivity, and (5) a desire for more connection (Miller & Stiver, 1991). Miller discussed the danger of meritocracy and disconnections and the tendency of traditional psychology to over-personalize problems (Jordan, 2008). She believed that the lack of connection is a source of psychological problems. Miller's work was the inspiration for Jordan's line of thinking. Jordan (2008) found that "The Five Good Things" were lacking in neglected and abused children who had experienced chronic disconnections. Instead, these children experienced (1) a drop in energy, (2) confusion, (3) a decreased sense of worth, (4) less productivity, and (5) withdrawal from all relationships. Individuals experiencing chronic disconnections described similar responses in therapy. Miller expressed concern about the dangers of chronic disconnections and asserted that people do not flourish by standing alone (Jordan, 2017). This highlights one of the ways in which Miller's ideas have been expanded and applied and evidence of Miller's impact on the field.

As the application of her relational approach evolved, Miller began incorporating more diverse voices and broader cultural contexts into the approach (Hartling, 2008). Since the fields of counseling and psychotherapy are normed by Eurocentric beliefs and values, intentionally seeking diversity was a departure from the theoretical work that had been done previously with White men. In addition to highlighting the voices of women, this diversification led to the challenging of inaccurate beliefs and ideas about other marginalized groups, as signaled by the name RCT. RCT offers a more balanced and accurate account of women and their contributions to the world than previous theories did (Jordan, 2008).

RCT posits that change is a bidirectional relational process of mutual development (Hartling, 2008). RCT focuses on the impact that power dynamics can have in a culture, within a family, and on a person's overall well-being. Disconnection and suffering can be caused by stratification, marginalization, and the exercise of dominance by one group over another, especially when that marginalized group is silenced, isolated, and shamed (Jordan, 2008, p. 4). Dangers of disconnection include emphasizing one's personal frailty rather than challenging the social conditions, stereotyping individuals of color and of different sexual orientations, and holding race- and class-based biases that prevent others' legitimate inclusion in pathways to social change (Jordan, 2008).

RCT highlights the social truth that dominant groups in a culture legitimize unequal relationships to obscure that truth and maintain the hierarchy (Hartling, 2008; Miller, 1986). RCT challenges the notion of meritocracy, such that at a societal level, those marginalized and positioned toward the bottom of the hierarchy are seen as failures, unmotivated, defective, and undeveloped (Jordan, 2017). These social constructs are psychologically harmful to individuals experiencing them and do not promote well-being. The goal, then, is to move beyond the traditional and limiting social paradigms and promote supportive relationships by focusing on the power of mutual respect and mutual learning that encourage ongoing growth and foster relationships (Jordan, 2008). The goal of therapy is to deepen the therapeutic relationship in order for the client to be able to deepen their relationships outside of therapy. The client's relational images are positive or negative expectations created by past relationships that in turn influence present and future relationships. The JBMTI continues to provide training and resources related to RCT, as do the many scholars who conduct research on the dynamics of power in therapy and the workplace, develop publications and training videos for therapists, and engage in the study of social neuroscience (Hartling, 2008). While initially challenged, the tenets of RCT have since been validated by modern neuroscience and are now embraced and supported by research.

Subversive Nature of Theory

While some critics feel Miller's work focuses a bit too narrowly on gender compared to other social differences, Zeedyk and Greenwood (2008) noted that Miller's greatest legacy is that she courageously sought to validate marginalized groups' personal experiences when it was not very popular to do so. Miller tried to remain true to the heart of feminism by advocating for social justice and equality for women everywhere, which was personal to her (Hartling, 2008; Zeedyk & Greenwood, 2008). Miller's work defied long-held myths of women's weakness by highlighting the social constructs put in place to mask the harmful impact of the powerful on vulnerable members of society (Hartling, 2008). In the United States and across the world, Miller's work created a new vision of womanhood and of mutuality in human relationships (Jordan, 2017; Zeedyk & Greenwood, 2008).

THEORIST BIOGRAPHY: KIMBERLÉ CRENSHAW

Kimberlé Williams Crenshaw was born 1959 in Canton, Ohio, to Walter Clarence Crenshaw Jr. and Marian Williams Crenshaw. Crenshaw is a legal scholar, civil rights activist, author, Black feminist, and a pioneer in two fields of study: critical race theory (CRT) and intersectionality. Crenshaw received her bachelor's degree in government and African studies from Cornell University (1981), a J.D. from Harvard Law School (1984), and an LL.M. from the University of Wisconsin (1985). Crenshaw has been a professor of law at the University of California, Los Angeles, since 1986 and at Columbia Law School since 1995. Her scholarly interests include law, civil rights, and CRT. She has received a number of prestigious awards and recognition, which include UCLA's graduating classes' Professor of the Year (1991 and 1994), a William H. Hastie fellowship while at the University of Wisconsin Law School, the Fulbright Chair for Latin America in Brazil (2007), an in-residence fellowship at the Center of Advanced Behavioral Studies at Stanford University (2009), Most Inspiring Feminist by *Ms. Magazine* (2015), one of the "Power 100" by *Ebony Magazine* (2015), Outstanding Scholar Award from the Fellows of the American Bar Foundation (2016), and the Gittler Prize (2017). She was also nominated for an Alphonse Fletcher fellowship (2008).

Throughout her career, Crenshaw has authored, coauthored, and edited numerous articles and chapters on CRT, intersectionality, race, gender, equality, and Black feminism. She is the cofounder and executive director of the African American Policy Forum (AAPF), which was established in 1996 to promote research-based strategies to advance social inclusion. Crenshaw travels the country speaking about and advocating for women's issues. Crenshaw is recognized as an influential thinker in several countries, including Brazil, France, Germany, Netherlands, Great Britain, and South Africa. Because of her global efforts, South Africa incorporated an equality clause in the nation's constitution (Gale, 2002). Additionally, Crenshaw has been instrumental in advocating for two antiviolence campaigns, most recently in 2020 "Why We Can't Wait" and "Say Her Name" in 2014. Crenshaw is considered one of the most sought-after speakers and foremost experts on race, gender, and various social justice issues.

Key Concepts and Utilization of Theory

People in the dominant culture have not considered the connection between sexism and other social categories such as race, class, and age. Individuals who have experienced oppression have always known, seen, and in many cases tried to articulate this connection, yet their voices were neither heard nor respected (Caldwell, 1995). Women such as Sojourner Truth (1797–1893), Susan B. Anthony (1820–1906), Anna Julia Cooper (1858–1964), and other notable women have spoken out and stood up for equality for centuries. Because of their efforts and the feminist movement, progress was made in the twentieth and early twenty-first centuries. However, another voice and perspective remained unheard regarding discriminatory practices within the social systems, and these were the voices of Black women (Coleman, 2019; Crenshaw, 1989).

In 1989, a vibrant, young legal scholar named Kimberlé Williams Crenshaw published the essay "Demarginalizing the Intersection of Race and Sex: A Black Feminist Critique of Antidiscrimination Doctrine, Feminist Theory, and Antiracist Politics," in which she described the multilayered discriminatory experiences of Black women as "intersectional." Based on her work with CRT, Crenshaw developed the concept of "intersectionality" to represent the unique and often complicated experiences of women of color, and specifically Black women, because of their race and gender (Coaston, 2019; Crenshaw, 1989). The courts at that time rejected Crenshaw's claim and considered discrimination to be a one-dimensional category with either race or gender as its basis (Coaston, 2019). The courts failed to consider that Black women are members of two marginalized groups, Black people and women.

The goal of Crenshaw's theory is to reframe society's understanding of how race and gender collectively have impacted the lives of women of color. The theory of intersectionality challenges the way "jurists, academics, and the media view issues of justice, prejudice, and identity" (Gale, 2002). Although the theory was publicly criticized during its embryotic stage, three decades later, Crenshaw's theory of intersectionality is considered by many scholars to be groundbreaking (Coleman, 2019). Today, the theory of intersectionality is commonly used and studied in disciplines including education, law, business, medicine, psychology, and sociology.

Crenshaw was instrumental in pioneering two schools of thought: CRT and intersectionality. The intellectual movement known as CRT was founded during the 1970s by several legal scholars to address the inequality among marginalized groups based on race, gender, class, and other social identities. The founders include Derrick Bell Jr., Alan Freeman, Charles Lawrence, Lani Guinier, Richard Delgado, Mai Matsuda, Patricia Williams, and Kimberlé Crenshaw (Allen, 2017). CRT emerged from the Critical Legal Studies (CSL) movement and was built upon Derrick Bell Jr.'s scholarship and critique of CSL's failure to adequately address racism or establish strategies for social change in light of the various forms of oppressive social structures and hierarchies that exist in the U.S. legal system (Allen, 2017; Caldwell, 1995; Griffin, 2010). CRT contested CSL's historical conceptions of the law as racially objective, neutral, color-blind, and apolitical (Caldwell, 1995). Based on the influence of the intellectual movement CRT, Crenshaw coined the term "intersectionality."

CRT's aim is to eliminate all forms of racism by exposing its Eurocentric epistemologies and how these racist practices are perpetuated today throughout history and within a social context (Griffin, 2010). Another goal of CRT is to address inequalities by engaging in social justice through activism (Delgado & Stefancic, 2017; Griffin, 2010). Griffin (2010) identified the seven tenets that many CRT scholars utilize: (1) interest convergence, (2) racism as every day, (3) color-blindness as insufficient, (4) race as a social construction, (5) Whiteness as property, (6) racialized narratives as significant and telling, and (7) racialized realities as contextual.

CRT scholars believe these tenets help elucidate the unique experiences of marginalized groups. *Interest convergence*, also referred to as *material determinism*, occurs when the interest to help people of color is more for one's personal advancement (i.e., material or psychological advancement) than the desire to eradicate the injustice. *Racism as every day* is what Delgado and Stefancic (2017) refer to as *ordinariness*, or the "the usual way society does business" (p. 8). *Ordinariness* occurs when society refuses to acknowledge the existence of racism (aka color-blindness), thus making racism difficult to address or cure (Delgado & Stefancic, 2017). Griffin (2010) argued that *color-blindness as insufficient* removes the mask or camouflage of racism and White privilege by revealing how those in power or dominant groups benefit greatly from the embrace of "colorblind" and "post-racial" discourse by maintaining the "status quo" (p. 4).

Race as a social construction, as described by Delgado and Stefancic (2017), suggests that races are categories that society creates and often manipulates as needed by focusing on common constructs within a race (i.e., physical) while ignoring the distinct higher-order traits (i.e., personality, intelligence, moral behavior). *Whiteness as property* is based on the premise that White or White-skinned individuals experienced privileges that other groups did not. White privilege was initiated and reinforced by laws before the U.S. legal system outlawed racial discrimination; however, it is still present today. *Racialized narratives as significant and telling* and *racialized realities as contextual* are critical components of CRT in that these tenets empowered marginalized groups to share their individual experiences where they own their stories of how race and racism have uniquely impacted their lives (Griffin, 2010). It is important to note that CRT is not about punishing White individuals or promoting Black superiority. Its focus is to raise individuals' social, economic, and political conscientiousness; eliminate all forms of social injustice; and promote activism.

The key concepts of the theory of intersectionality. While many of its concepts have their underpinnings in the work of Black feminists, the intersectional framework is designed to serve as a lens by which society pays attention to individuals who are marginally oppressed. CRT and the theory of intersectionality challenge the historical systems that reinforce bias and discriminatory practices in all forms. The core tenets of intersectionality focus on addressing the interlocking systems of oppression and promoting the need for structural-level changes (Rosenthal, 2016). The key concept of *interlocking systems of oppression* are multiple systems of oppression that are simultaneously connected among social categories, interpersonal interactions or stigmas, and societal systems. The term "interlocking" is also used to describe the crossroads of multiple oppressions (Marecek, 2016).

Social categories are often referred to as intersecting categories. Many scholars believe that it is these social or intersecting categories "upon which such systems are built" (Marecek, 2016). Social categories initially focused on race, gender, and class; now other categories such as nationality, age, and sexuality are often considered (Marecek, 2016). Another key concept is *structural-level changes*. Structural-level changes focus on the need to dismantle and eradicate harmful societal structures, which are often historical practices that reinforce forms of privilege for some and forms of oppression for others through laws, policies, stereotypical media representations, unemployment, various forms of segregation, and poverty (Rosenthal, 2016).

Crenshaw initially described intersectionality using Black women as the prototype. The theory has since been expanded to include women of all races and ethnicities. Intersectionality has created a platform that allows marginalized groups of various races, classes, gender identifications, and sexuality to have a voice that they were not allowed decades before. Because of intersectionality's increasing popularity, some scholars are concerned about departing from its original intent, while other critics argue that the theory has already mutated and been corrupted (Gillborn, 2015; Marecek, 2016). Like CRT, intersectionality continues to evolve as scholars and researchers find unique ways to advocate for social change. Howard and Navarro (2016) described CRT as a transformative, methodological, and theoretical construct particularly in the area of education.

CRT and intersectionality have been widely used among various cultures and disciplines. Various scholars in fields ranging from communication, education, political science, to sociology all utilize CRT. CRT allows for flexibility when adhering to the use of its tenets. CRT scholars have found many of tenets to be helpful to them in their research. For example, Allen (2017) found educators are able to examine color-blindness in curriculum, pedagogy, teaching, and learning through the CRT lens in order to make changes in the educational system; researchers have also found CRT to be a helpful tool when transforming current school practices.

Intersectionality is more of a theoretical framework than it is the traditional testable form of theory found in the social sciences and academia (Bowleg, 2012). While many scholars have used some variation of intersectionality in their research, the framework primarily has been used as an analytical tool to identify forms of inequality and connections to interlocking systems of oppression in disciplines such as sociology, psychology, education, and public health (Bowleg, 2012; Rosenthal, 2016).

Subversive Nature of Theory

Crenshaw's work with CRT and her theory of intersectionality has had a significant impact in the United States and across the world. With the help of sociologist Patricia Collins, who has contributed to the expansion of the theory of intersectionality and its applications, many disciplines have embraced this theory as a lens with which scholars study, interact, and relate to different social identities. Intersectionality is undoubtedly influencing clinical practices, instructional practices, and curriculum pedagogy in schools in both undergraduate and graduate programs. It is also impacting how research is used and analyzed from a critical race paradigm. While intersectionality has its advantages, it is not devoid of limitations. Scholars must be careful not to deviate from its original intent, which is to eliminate all forms of harmful social structures. While there are multilevel approaches to intervention, intersectionality, like CRT, is rooted in activism that promotes social justice and equality (Rosenthal, 2016).

Both Miller and Crenshaw homed in on culture as a necessary context for understanding women's experiences. Some of the theorists mentioned in the previous chapters did this, too. However, Miller and Crenshaw focused on culture to a greater extent. Miller provided a perspective of our social and political structures in a way that helped men and women understand how characteristics attributed to men are preferred, thus providing the structures to keep men holding power and privilege, maintaining the status quo. Crenshaw took that a step farther to identify not only gender but also how oppression is multiplied when women belong to a gender subordinate group and also a racial subordinate group, such as Black, Indigenous, and People of Color experience in the U.S. Miller and Crenshaw theorized a new and intersectional understanding of the systemic and oppressive lenses through which people may viewed and the subsequent impact on mental health, permanently changing counseling and psychological theories.

REFERENCES

Allen, M. (2017). The relevance of critical race theory: Impact on students of color. *Urban Education Research & Policy Annuals*, *5*(1), 1–9. https://journals.uncc.edu/urbaned/article/view/575

Bowleg, L. (2012). The problem with the phrase *women and minorities*: Intersectionality—an important theoretical framework for public health. *American Journal of Public Health*, *102*(7), 1267–1273. doi:10.2105/AJPH.2012.300750

Caldwell, V. F. (1995). Critical race theory: The key writings that formed the movement. Edited by Kimberlé Williams Crenshaw et al. *Columbia Law Review*, *96*(5), 1363–1374. https://www.jstor.org/stable/1123408

Coaston, J. (2019). The intersectionality wars. *Vox*. https://www.vox.com/the-highlight/2019/5/20/18542843/intersectionality-conservatism-law-race-gender-discrimination

Coleman, A. L. (2019). What's intersectionality? Let these scholars explain the theory and its history. *Time Magazine*. https://time.com/5560575/intersectionality-theory/

Crenshaw, K. (1989). Demarginalizing the intersection of race and sex: A black feminist critique of antidiscrimination doctrine, feminist theory and antiracist politics. *University of Chicago Legal Forum*, 139–168. https://chicagounbound.uchicago.edu/uclf/vol1989/iss1/8

Delgado, R., & Stefancic, J. (2017). *Critical Race Theory* (3rd edition). New York University Press.

Gillborn, D. (2015). Intersectionality, critical race theory, and the primacy of racism: Race, class, gender, and disability in education. *Qualitative Inquiry*, *21*(3), 277–287. doi:10.1177/1077800414557827

Griffin, R. A. (2010). Critical race theory as a means to deconstruct, recover and evolve in communication studies. *Communication Law Review*, *10*(1), 1–9. http://www.commlawreview.org/Archives/CLRv10i1/PDFs/Critical_Race_Theory_as_a_Means_to_Deconstruct_Recover_and_Evolve_in_Communication_Studies.pdf

Hartling, L. (2008). Jean Baker Miller: Living in connection. *Feminism & Psychology*, *18*(3), 326–335. doi:10.1177/0959353508092085

Howard, T. C., & Navarro, O. (2016). Critical race theory 20 years later: Where do we go from here? *Urban Education*, *51*(3), 253–273. doi:10.1177/0042085915622541

Jean Baker Miller Training Institute (JBMTI). (2019). The development of relational-cultural theory beginnings: Self-in-relation. *Wellesley Centers for Women*. https://www.wcwonline.org/JBMTI-Site/the-development-of-relational-cultural-theory

Jordan, J. V. (2008). Recent developments in relational-cultural theory. *Women & Therapy*, *31*(2–4), 1–4. doi:10.1080/02703140802145540

Jordan, J. V. (2017) Jean Baker Miller, MD: Visionary pragmatist. *Women & Therapy*, *40*(3–4), 260–274. doi:10.1080/02703149.2017.1241568

"Kimberle Williams Crenshaw." Gale Biography Online Collection, Gale, 2002. Gale In Context: Biography, https://link.gale.com/apps/doc/K1650002325/BIC?u=vic_liberty&sid=BIC&xid=318f37cc

Marecek, J. (2016). Invited reflection: Intersectionality theory and feminist psychology. *Psychology of Women Quarterly*, *40*(2), 177–181. doi:10.1177/0361684316641090

Miller, J. B. (1986). *Toward a New Psychology of Women* (2nd edition). Beacon Press.

Miller, J. B. (1988). *Connections, Disconnections, and Violations* (Work in Progress No. 33). Stone Center Working Paper Series. https://www.wcwonline.org/pdf/previews/preview_33sc.pdf

Miller, J. B., & Stiver, I. R. (1991). *A Relational Reframing of Therapy* (Work in Progress No. 52). Stone Center Working Paper Series. https://www.wcwonline.org/pdf/previews/preview_52sc.pdf

Rosenthal, L. (2016). Incorporating intersectionality into psychology: An opportunity to promote social justice and equity. *American Psychologist*, *71*(6), 474–485. doi:10.1037/a0040323

Zeedyk, M., & Greenwood, R. (2008). Reflections on the work of feminist theorist Jean Baker Miller. *Feminism & Psychology*, *18*(3), 321–325. doi:10.1177/0959353508092084

Chapter 7

Children and Family Systems Theorists

Women have transformed theories of counseling and psychotherapy with their focus on children and family systems. As covered in chapter 2, the idea of providing counseling to children started in the late 1920s with Anna Freud and Melanie Klein, who applied the principles of psychoanalysis to children. In the 1940s, Virginia Axline (1911–1988) expanded on this work to pioneer the use of play therapy. Current practices in play therapy are still largely based on Axline's work. In the mid-twentieth century, a shift occurred from a belief that behavior originates with the individual to systemic theories, which conceptualize of human behavior as behavior that is created and maintained by relationships. While traditional mental health perspectives posit that behavior originates with the individual, systemic theories provide the guiding principles within the professions of family counseling and therapy. Virginia Satir (1916–1988) is one of the few women who developed a theoretical approach and a model with her own name, the Virginia Satir model. Satir emphasized the process of change and considered experiences, interpersonal connections, and perceptions that impact people at an emotional level. Axline and Satir are two women pioneers who made significant contributions to therapy focusing on children and families.

THEORIST BIOGRAPHY: VIRGINIA AXLINE

Virginia Mae Axline was born in Fort Wayne, Indiana, in 1911, but she grew up in Columbus, Ohio. Virginia passed away in Ohio in 1988 at the age of seventy-seven and was buried next to her mother, father, and older sister. Axline worked as a schoolteacher in Ohio for several years before she attended graduate school at Ohio State University.

Key Concepts and Utilization of Theory

While there, she began to collaborate with Carl Rogers. In 1945 Rogers opened the University of Chicago Counseling Center where for three years, Axline was one of his research associates. During this time, Axline began to develop her own approach to counseling children. In 1947 Axline wrote and published the book *Play Therapy*, which represented the launch of her theory of child psychotherapy. In her book she outlined eight basic principles of play therapy that have stood the passage of time as a method for treating children. In 1950 Axline completed her doctorate of education at Columbia University Teachers College. Virginia taught at the New York University School of Medicine and School of Education in addition to Columbia University Teachers College. She remained as faculty for several years before returning to Ohio where she taught at Ohio State University and maintained a private practice. In 1964 she wrote *Dibs in Search of Self*, a book that provides details of her clinical work including verbatim transcripts of weekly sessions. The book documents the application of Axline's nondirective approach to play therapy and the transformation of a silent five-year-old boy named Dibs. The book became popular; however, Axline preferred a quiet life and declined invitations to be in the spotlight.

Axline began to explore nonverbal therapeutic play with children while studying under Rogers. At the same time that Rogers was developing his person-centered approach to working with adults, Axline was incorporating similar principles into her work with children. Initially known as nondirective play therapy and then later as child-centered play therapy (CCPT), Axline's approach is grounded in genuine warmth, empathy, and unconditional positive regard. Fundamental to Axline's theory is the belief that children naturally move toward growth and development if provided an environment that is warm and supportive. She believed that children communicate thoughts and express feelings through their use of toys. The goal is to facilitate healing and change, both psychological and behavioral.

The locus of control resides within the child; therefore, change must originate within the child. The therapist creates an environment in which the child feels safe enough to express their feelings. This process facilitates congruence and movement for the child to make changes that grow toward self-actualization, which is a unified, organized, holistic, and congruent expression of the child's self.

Axline identified the following eight core principles for working with children in her book *Play Therapy* as explained in table 7.1:

Table 7.1 Axline's Eight Core Principles for Play Therapy with Children

1. *The therapist must develop a warm, friendly relationship with the child, in which good rapport is established as soon as possible.*

At face value this appears simple; however, it can be particularly challenging with young children for whom the therapist is a stranger. A therapist builds rapport through nonjudgmental, unconditional positive regard; sensitively validates feelings; and responds empathetically to the needs of the child. As part of this principle, the therapist establishes consistent rules to create emotional and physical safety and allows the child to be self-directed. Axline worked with children alone; she did not believe it was necessary to work with parents in order to help a child. She set a boundary with parents such that they were never allowed to enter the playroom. It may take more time for the therapist to develop rapport with older children who have issues with trust. As trust is built within the therapeutic relationship, a child gains a sense of mastery and trust within their core self.

2. *The therapist accepts the child exactly as they are.*

This means that the therapist is very attuned to how a child may be feeling but does not take care of or redirect the child who is experiencing difficult emotions to help them feel better. Instead the therapist may make an observational statement to help a child identify and label their thoughts and feelings. The underlying assumption is that children are doing exactly what they need to do in order to work through their own problems, and the therapist maintains a nonjudgmental stance except in establishing rules for safety.

3. *The therapist establishes a feeling of permissiveness in the relationship so that the child feels free to express his feelings completely.*

Children lead the sessions and the therapist grants permission using tone, facial expressions, and body language. The therapist does not provide any direction, thus communicating to children that they have the freedom to spontaneously express any thought or feeling they have without a hint of leading by the therapist. The therapist needs to preserve a nonjudgmental stance and avoid communicating expectations through negative or positive messages. Though this stance may be difficult for the therapist to maintain, the therapist must be careful to avoid providing encouragement or praise, asking questions or giving prompts, or providing direction. Patience on the part of the therapist is crucial for the child to express their feelings and issues at a comfortable pace, which ultimately helps the child learn to navigate thoughts, feelings, and behavior.

4. *The therapist is alert to recognize the feelings the child is expressing and reflects those feelings back to him in such a manner that he gains insight into his behavior.*

One of the core skills of the therapist is to engage in active, empathetic listening to communicate to children that the therapist is aware of and interested in their play and ideas. Unlike mechanical parroting or analysis, empathetic listening is a gentle and nonintrusive skill by which the therapist identifies, accepts, and labels emotions nonjudgmentally. This may involve the therapist making behavioral observations and connecting feelings with a child's play behavior. The therapist needs to use this strategy regardless of the child's particular emotion. Empathetic listening requires the therapist to have an awareness of the child's emotions, as indicated by the child's facial expressions, tone, and body language. Responses occur frequently when a therapist is working to develop rapport and create a safe environment; they taper off in the later stages of therapy.

(*Continued*)

Table 7.1 Axline's Eight Core Principles for Play Therapy with Children (*Continued*)

5. *The therapist maintains a deep respect for the child's ability to solve his own problems if given an opportunity to do so. The responsibility to make choices and institute change is the child's.*
There is a foundational belief that children can solve their own problems. The therapist needs to demonstrate this belief through permissiveness, acceptance, and observations. The therapist needs to be attuned to the individual needs of a child and respond therapeutically. For instance, the therapist may need to avoid helping a child who is frustrated or aiding a child who has asked for help. The child senses the therapist's trust in them, which ultimately facilitates the child's internalization of trust and self-acceptance. Using play, children learn that they are responsible for themselves and their behavior. This means that the therapist demonstrates respect for the child's decisions in the playroom and recognizes these decisions are necessary for the child to develop mastery over themselves and the environment.
6. *The therapist does not attempt to direct the child's actions or conversation in any manner. The child leads the way; the therapist follows.*
After the therapist communicates the rules for safety, the child has the responsibility to decide on their behavior in the playroom. Children are very aware of adult expectations, and they pay close attention to nonverbal communications. It can be uncomfortable for a child to take the lead before they have developed trust in the therapist. The therapist can facilitate trust by adhering to the nondirection principle. This is often a list of activities to avoid, such as making judgments; teaching, giving suggestions, praise, or criticism; interpreting and evaluating; and asking questions. Avoiding engaging in these activities communicates to the child that the therapist believes in an innate drive toward development and trusts and respects the child's ability to solve their own problems. The therapist becomes a human mirror, providing observations and feeling reflections to demonstrate their connection with and trust in the child's learning process.
7. *The therapist does not attempt to hurry the therapy along. It is a gradual process and is recognized as such by the therapist.*
Children are growing and learning to become adults, which is a process that takes approximately eighteen years. Children are learning about themselves and others and how to navigate their environments. Each child learns at their own pace. Therapists accept and respect each child's developmental pace and are patient with their process. Therapists communicate that there is no hurry because the child leads the sessions.
8. *The therapist establishes only those limitations that are necessary to anchor the therapy to the world of reality and to make the child aware of his responsibility in the relationship.*
Limits are crucial to ensure safety in the playroom. There are not very many limits within the playroom, but those that do exist are very important. Children depend on adults to establish limits, and through limits and consequences, children come to learn self-control and appropriate behaviors. Children are not able to establish rapport with or trust adults who do not establish and maintain clear limits for safety.

In her detailed book, *Dibs in Search of Self*, Axline identifies and explains the application of her eight principles and the methods she used to interact with Dibs. The book has become one of the most influential books in the field of play therapy and a part of the curriculum at many colleges and universities. CCPT has been used effectively in a variety of cultural contexts. Axline's theoretical foundation of growth and development toward a healthy self transcends cultural boundaries to focus on the human condition as evidenced in children.

Through her eight core concepts, Axline catapulted play therapy into a theoretical idea of its own and influenced many other therapists. Violet Oaklander extended Axline's concepts by incorporating Gestalt therapy into play therapy. The founder of Play Therapy International (PTI), Mark Burnes, integrated all of Axline's approaches into his work with children, ultimately producing the world's first standards in play therapy training and education. CCPT is now one of the most thoroughly researched theoretical models of play therapy in the world.

Subversive Nature of Theory

Virginia Axline was a student of Carl Rogers, and her work was influenced by his. However, she did not remain under his tutelage as would have been customary for a woman to do during this time in history. She independently published her work and developed her ideas alone. It was not her strong personality or connections with others that propelled her work forward. Rather, it is the work itself that will keep her name forever inscribed in history as the theorist who developed the first nondirective play therapy. Axline's theories continue to provide the foundation for play therapy throughout the world.

THEORIST BIOGRAPHY: VIRGINIA SATIR

Virginia Satir (née Pagenkopf) was born on June 26, 1916, in Niellsville, Wisconsin, and passed away on September 10, 1988, in Menlo Park, California, at the age of seventy-two. Satir was raised on a farm with her three younger brothers and one younger sister in a second-generation German-American family. She was curious and had a love for knowledge. At the age of five, she foreshadowed her career exploring human behavior by saying that when she grew up, she was going to be a children's detective investigating parents (Satir, 1988). She was very bright, reading by age three, graduating from high school at age fifteen, and graduating from the University of Wisconsin in 1936 at age twenty with a bachelor's degree in education.

She became a public schoolteacher and at that time conceptualized the reciprocal relationship between students' problems and their families (Suarez, 2012). Beginning in 1937 Satir took classes in social work for three summers at Northwestern University in Chicago, Illinois; she then enrolled full-time at the University of Chicago. Satir completed her coursework in 1943, but her master's degree in social work was conferred by the University of Chicago School of Social Services Administration five years later in 1948, once she had completed her thesis (Suarez, 2012).

Satir married Gordon Rodgers in 1941. Rogers left her a few months after they were married to fight in World War II and they divorced in 1949. Virginia Satir married Norman Satir in 1951, and they divorced in 1957. When Satir was asked to explain her marriages and divorces, she said that she would have done a lot of things differently and described her relationship hindsight as "wonderful for writing Ph.D. papers but not very good for life" (King, 1989, as cited in Suarez, 2012.)

Introduction to Theory

Satir accomplished much during her career. She began as a schoolteacher and developed into a well-known international trainer. Satir began working while in high school during the Great Depression and continued during college to support herself. Her professional clinical work began at the Chicago Home for Girls and the Institute for Juvenile Research in Chicago. In 1951 Satir began to focus on working with families rather than individuals. At the Illinois State Psychiatric Institute of Chicago, Satir developed her first family therapy training program. In 1959 Satir moved to Palo Alto, California, where she co-founded the experientially based Mental Research Institute (MRI). In 1962 the MRI was awarded a National Institute of Mental Health grant through which Satir developed the first formal family therapy training program. Satir was the director of this program until 1966. Satir began visiting the Esalen Institute in Big Sur, California, where she discovered meditation and bodywork and explored new ideas. In 1970 Satir organized the Beautiful People network, which later became known as the International Human Learning Resources Network. In 1977 she founded the Avanta Network, which was renamed the Virginia Satir Global Network in 2010.

Satir published her first book, *Conjoint Family Therapy*, in 1964. Other books include *Self-Esteem* (1970), *Peoplemaking* (1972), *Making Contact* (1976), *Your Many Faces* (1978), and *The New Peoplemaking* (1988). She coauthored other books and articles throughout her career and developed many training groups. Satir received awards and honors too numerous to detail. The highlights are that Satir was invited to be a member of the Council of Elders, a select group of world citizens who meet with Nobel Laureates for World Peace; was appointed to the Steering Committee of the International Family Therapy Association; and was a member of the Advisory Board for the National Council for Self-Esteem. She became a diplomat of the Academy of Certified Social Workers and was granted an honorary doctorate from the University of Wisconsin, Madison. Satir was an innovator in family therapy until her death in 1988 from pancreatic cancer. Satir Centers and Institutes continue to operate all over the world.

Key Concepts and Utilization of Theory

Satir is considered a founder in family therapy. One of her statements is representative of her many conceptual contributions: "The family is a microcosm. By knowing how to heal the family, I know how to heal the world." Satir's theoretical approach was influenced by the humanistic movement, general systems theory, and cybernetics. Satir's work is sometimes conceptualized as experiential, integrative, developmental, and spiritual, traits that set it apart from the focus on objectivity at the time. At the core of her philosophy is the belief that individuals are capable of continued growth, change, and new understandings in order to fulfill their potential. She placed an emphasis on communication, the influence of the family of origin, and the importance of revising any negative impact on the current family system.

Virginia Satir model. Virginia Satir is one of the few women who developed a theoretical approach and a model that bears her own name. Satir's model is known by several different names, including the conjoint family therapy model, human growth model, human validation model, Satir family therapy model, Satir model, and Satir process model. The Virginia Satir model is grounded in instinctive interventions without structured techniques. She also developed the mandala as a schema that organizes the multiple different influences of human experience into eight different levels: the physical domain, the emotional domain, the sensual domain, the interactional domain, the nutritional domain, the contextual domain, and the spiritual domain (Satir & Baldwin, 1983). Her model involves experiences, interpersonal connections, and perceptions that impact individuals on an emotional level. The therapist's role is to act as a flexible and spontaneous facilitator who is fully present and uses immediacy to influence change. In order to facilitate effectively, the Satir model provides space for reflections on oneself and others. Satir said, "Our biggest problem as human beings is not knowing that we don't know" (Suarez, 2012). Satir believed that therapists need to engage with their inner selves in order to become more integrated with their external presentation, which positively impacts their work with couples and families.

A primary concept of the Satir model is that self-esteem is one of the most fundamental functions of families that affects congruent communication and coping skills. There is a belief that each person in the family is needed and makes a difference. Satir believed that individuals in families with healthy self-esteem can clearly and congruently present their position, ask for and provide clarification, openly receive feedback, and grow. Healthy family members congruently communicate support of other family members' growth, and the family environment fosters taking risks, expressing feelings, and expressing differences. Satir believed there is an exponential relationship between indirect communication and dysfunction. Dysfunctional families often engage in indirect methods of communication that include misinterpretations, assumptions, and generalizations. Families with maladaptive self-esteem do not value an individual sense of self-worth or the fulfillment of potential for personal growth. Individuals with low self-esteem do not value themselves, do not communicate support for the growth of others, create dysfunctional environments, and respond to others in unhealthy and maladaptive ways. Families with low self-esteem have poor communication and maladaptive coping skills that are passed on to future generations unless redirected upward to foster the natural innate growth process.

The Satir model is considered a growth model, and Satir believed that individuals and families already possess all they need to grow. Satir believed that one of the greatest gifts she could receive from anyone was to be seen, heard, understood and touched by them. Therefore, she also believed that the greatest gift she could give to another was to see, hear, understand, and touch that person. Satir believed that by doing so, contact had been made. In the Satir model, the client is responsible for change that is facilitated through the therapist's use of self. Satir held a deep belief that humans are all spiritual beings. She believed in a universal life force of energy that was both unique to each person and at the same time connected with all. Satir believed that connecting with one's spiritual energy leads to wholeness and one's best self. In contrast, disconnection from spiritual energy and the suppression of feelings comprise the foundation of emotional pain, broken relationships, and behavioral dysfunction. The goal is to develop a therapeutic alliance such that clients feel safe to express deeply suppressed emotions that block natural growth and fulfillment. The therapeutic methods the Satir model uses to achieve this goal are often experiential, as Satir believed that experiential awareness important for growth. The methods include sculpting, psychodrama, family reconstruction, role play, art therapy, the use of triads and metaphors, the teaching and modeling of effective communication, and the therapist's use of self. Therapy involves encouraging the client to lean into difficult feelings, to accept the present, to connect to their spiritual energy, and to open their hearts to others.

Satir's overarching mantra was "Peace within, peace between, peace among" (Suarez, 2012).

One of Satir's most novel ideas at the time was that a client's presenting problem is usually a surface problem and how the person copes is the real problem. The Satir model uses the iceberg as a metaphor to illustrate the complexity of humans (Lee, 2002). The iceberg metaphor is used to suggest that individuals are holistic, multilayered, interdependent systems. The tip of the iceberg above the waterline is interpersonal communication stances of behavior and coping. These are but a small part of the whole person; most of the person is found deep below the surface. Just below the waterline is the intrapsychic dimension, which includes constructs of feelings, feelings about feelings, perceptions and beliefs, and expectations of self and others. These constructs create barriers of connection to one's universal life energy. Following the Satir model, therapists use experiential interventions to unblock the constructs in this domain. The therapist facilitates the client's experiential awareness of past feelings and unmet expectations in order for the client to process them and develop new congruent interpersonal choices.

The widest part of the iceberg is the universal spiritual dimension, or what Satir referred to as life force. The spiritual dimension includes a person's yearnings, including love, acceptance, belonging, creativity, connection, and freedom. The deepest layer of the iceberg is identified as the self that Satir called the "I am." Satir described this part of the person as the soul, life force, essence, and core being. Using the iceberg metaphor, the therapist highlights for the client how change in one aspect of the system becomes a catalyst for changes in all others. The goal is for every client to have open congruent connection between the deepest level of the universal spiritual dimension, through the intrapsychic domain to the interpersonal communication and coping behaviors above the waterline.

Although the Satir model appears to adhere to the Western value of individualism, this model is based on universal human qualities and resources and can be applied to other cultures. Therapists using this model must be culturally sensitive because change in an individual must align with that individual's cultural values. A client who is situated in a highly collectivist culture will not be able to sustain individual change if the therapist focuses only on the individual, overlooking cultural expectations and values. Additionally, the experiential nature of therapy and the focus on personal feelings may be very difficult for a client from a nondemonstrative culture that values keeping feelings inside. However, the Satir model conceptualizes individuals from a systems perspective, such as within the context of family. The Satir model is sensitive to cultural values and is applicable to all human communication and growth, whether that growth is conceptualized as occurring within a person, a family, a community, or a company. This is evidenced by the international acceptance of the Satir model and the establishment of training groups around the world in Asia, Central and Latin America, Eastern and Western Europe, and Russia.

Subversive Nature of Theory

When Virginia was a child growing up, people of German ancestry were viewed with suspicion as possible German spies. They were often asked to prove their loyalty to the United States. At one time Satir indicated she had issues with her heritage and would not travel to Germany for many years. The context in which Satir was raised contributed to the development of her personal strength and may have prepared her for working in the male-dominated psychoanalytic and psychotherapy communities. Even though the underlying conceptualizations of general systems theory and cybernetics are systemic and contributed to the development of Satir's theory, they are very scientific and structured. Additionally, much of the psychoanalytical and cognitive theories of the time did not require introspection on the part of the therapist because of the aspirational notion of therapist neutrality and objectivity.

Satir tried to engage with clients in this way, seeing only individual clients, but she found this to be uncomfortable and incongruent. Satir did not follow the scientific norms of her time, significantly diverging from theories that focused on observational external objectivity to develop her own theory that embraced unseen, subjective intuition and spirituality. Satir was intuitive and spoke of people as sacred. Her idea of a connection with a universal life force aligned more with religious than with scientific communities. This directional change was like disembarking from a train to forge a completely different path in a jungle with a machete. Given the context of the time, it was not surprising that Satir encountered resistance to her theory and shifted her efforts away from the field to travel and lecturing.

Satir's prominence throughout the world, not just her ideas, but her as a person differs from many of the other women in this book. One can only speculate as to why she is often found or listed in historical textbooks on counseling and psychological theories. Other women theorist were often invisible as people even when their ideas were utilized. It may have been personal characteristics such as her physical presence, large stature, or extroverted nature. Satir seems to be an outlier in our study of women theorists, and we look forward to discovering what enabled her to develop an international career while other women could not. We may need to wait until more women theorists in counseling and psychotherapy have similar success to discover the common themes.

REFERENCES

Axline, V. M. (1947/1969). *Play Therapy*. Ballantine Books.

Axline, V. M. (1964/1986). *Dibs in Search of Self*. Ballantine Books.

Baggerly, J., & Parker, M. (2005). Child-centered group play therapy with African American boys at the elementary school level. *Journal of Counseling & Development*, *83*(4), 387–396. doi:10.1002/j.1556-6678.2005.tb00360.x

Banmen, A., & Banmen, J. (eds.). (1991). *Meditations of Virginia Satir*. Science and Behavior Books.

Banmen, J. (2002). Introduction: Virginia Satir today. *Contemporary Family Therapy*, *24*(1), 3–5. doi:10.1023/A:1014302720012

Banmen, J. (2002). The Satir model: Yesterday and today. *Contemporary Family Therapy*, *24*(1), 7–22. doi:10.1023/A:1014365304082

Carlock, C. J. (2013). A "Wheel of Resources" for emergency first responders. *Satir Journal of Counselling and Family Therapy*, *1*, 1–9. https://journals.uvic.ca/index.php/satir/article/view/11561

Chang, C. Y., Ritter, K. B., & Hays, D. G. (2005). Multicultural trends and toys in play therapy. *International Journal of Play Therapy*, *14*(2), 69–85. doi:10.1037/h0088903

Cheung, G., & Chan, C. (2002). The Satir model and cultural sensitivity: A Hong Kong reflection. *Contemporary Family Therapy*, *24*(1), 199–215. doi:10.1023/A:1014338025464

Davis, E. S., & Pereira, J. K. (2014). Child-centered play therapy: A creative approach to culturally competent counseling. *Journal of Creativity in Mental Health*, *9*(2), 262–274. doi:10.1080/15401383.2014.892863

Erker, J. (2017). A summary of a qualitative study of Satir family therapy: Theoretical and practical developments over the past 30 years. *Satir International Journal*, *5*(1), 76–81. https://journals.uvic.ca/index.php/satir/article/view/17876

Garza, Y., & Bratton, S. C. (2005). School-based child-centered play therapy with Hispanic children: Outcomes and cultural consideration. *International Journal of Play Therapy*, *14*(1), 51–80. doi:10.1037/h0088896

Haber, R. (2002). Virginia Satir: An integrated, humanistic approach. *Contemporary Family Therapy*, *24*(1), 23–34. doi:10.1023/A:1014317420921

Innes, M. (2002). Satir's therapeutically oriented educational process: A critical appreciation. *Contemporary Family Therapy*, *24*(1), 35–56. doi:10.1023/A:1014369504991

Landreth, G. (2012). *Play therapy: The Art of the Relationship* (3rd edition). Routledge.

Lee, B. K. (2002). Congruence in Satir's model: Its spiritual and religious significance. *Contemporary Family Therapy*, *24*(1), 57–78. doi:10.1023/A:1014390009534

Li, Y., & Lou, V. W. Q. (2013). Applying the Satir model of counseling in mainland China: Illustrated with 20 case sessions. *Satir Journal of Counseling and Family Therapy*, *1*, 18–39. https://journals.uvic.ca/index.php/satir/article/view/11559

Lum, W. (2002). The use of self of the therapist. *Contemporary Family Therapy*, *24*(1), 181–197. doi:10.1023/A:1014385908625

Pelak, D. (2016). A recursive frame analysis of Satir through the biopsychosocial lens. *The Qualitative Report, 21*(6), 996–1015. https://nsuworks.nova.edu/tqr/vol21/iss6/1

Play Therapy International South Africa. (2013). Axline principles of play therapy. http://www.saplaytherapyinternational.org.za/axlineprinciples.html

Pope, V. T., & Lawrence, C. (2017). Virginia Satir model. In J. Carlson & S. B. Dermer (eds.), *The SAGE Encyclopedia of Marriage, Family, and Couples Counseling* (pp. 248–253). Sage Publications, Inc.

Ray, D. (2011). *Advanced Play Therapy: Essential Conditions, Knowledge, and Skill for Child Practice*. Routledge.

Satir, V. (1964/1967/1983). *Conjoint Family Therapy* (3rd edition). Science and Behavior Books.

Satir, V. (1970/1995/2001). *Self-esteem*. Celestial Arts.

Satir, V. (1972/1990). *Peoplemaking*. Souvenir Press.

Satir, V. (1976). *Making Aontact*. Celestial Arts.

Satir, V. (1978). *Your Many Faces*. Celestial Arts.

Satir, V. (1988). *The New Peoplemaking*. Science and Behavior Books.

Satir, V., & Baldwin, M. (1983). *Satir Step by Step: A Guide to Creating Change in Families*. Science and Behavior Books.

Satir, V., Bandler, R., & Grinder, J. (1976). *Changing with Families*. Science and Behavior Books.

Satir, V., Banmen, J., Gerber, J., & Gomori, M. (1991). *The Satir Model: The Family and Beyond*. Science and Behavior Books.

Satir, V., Stachowiak, J., & Taschman, H. A. (1994). *Helping Families to Change*. Jason Aronson.

Suarez, M. (2012). *Who Virginia Satir Was and Why She Mattered*. Retrieved from https://web.archive.org/web/20120425040023/http://satirglobal.org/about-virginia-satir/

Taylor, G. (2002). Family reconstruction. *Contemporary Family Therapy, 24*(1), 129–138 doi:10.1023/A:1014329823646

VanFleet, R., Sywulak, A. E., & Sniscak, C. C. (2010). *Child-Centered Play Therapy*. Guilford Press.

Conclusion

Other Women Theorists and Themes

As you read this book, you learned about some of the women who helped further and expand others' theories or created psychotherapy theories of their own. The women included in the preceding chapters are not an exhaustive list of all women who have created theories of mental health and wellness. Rather, we chose women whose theories were some of the most well established and relevant to the fields of counseling and psychotherapy. We found similarities and themes with the lives and circumstances of the women theorists covered in this book. Additionally, there are other women who could have been included but were not. We provide a more thorough list of women and their accomplishments in counseling and psychotherapy below. Some of these women did not create theories, though the importance of their work merits their inclusion in this book.

OTHER WOMEN THEORISTS

Theodora Mead Abel

Theodora Mead Abel (1899–1998) was born in Newport, Rhode Island. Abel was one of the first psychologists to assert culture was an imperative component in therapy. Beginning in 1947, Abel worked with and studied various cultures such as the Chinese, Mexican, Syrian, and French cultures. She utilized this work in the 1960s and established one of the earliest training programs in cross-cultural psychotherapy. She went on to use cross-cultural family therapy techniques with Mescalero, Jicarilla Apaches, and Navajo Native Americans in New Mexico. Two of her contributions to the fields of counseling and psychotherapy are revealing the "culture-boundedness of all mental and personality tests" and the "impact of cultural beliefs and modes of behavior on various aspects of psychotherapy" (Ware, 2005, p. 4).

Louise Bates Ames

Louise Bates Ames (1908–1996) was born in Portland, Maine. Ames's work centered on child development and, perhaps most notably, contributed to the phrase "the terrible twos." Her most radical work, however, was in the 1940s; she stressed the importance of parents accepting unconventional child gender variances.

Carolyn Attneave

Carolyn Attneave (1920–1992) was born in Texas. She was of Scandinavian and Delaware Native American descent. She was passionate about providing mental health care to Native Americans and worked with at least seven tribes while living in Oklahoma. She utilized her cross-culture competence to focus on network therapy, which emphasizes the need for community, family, and personal networks in mental health treatment.

Martha Bernal

Martha Bernal (1931–2001) was born in San Antonio, Texas. In 1962 she became the first Mexican American to earn a doctorate in clinical psychology in the United States. Her research focused on minority mental health and the best strategies for training minorities in psychology programs. She established the National Latino Psychological Association.

Mamie Phipps Clark

Mamie Phipps Clark (1917–1983) was born in Hot Spring, Arkansas. Clark was the first African American woman to enter and complete a psychology doctoral program at Columbia University. She was the twenty-second African American to obtain a psychology doctorate in the United States. Clark is best known for her work on children's racial concepts and the utilization of dolls to assess the internalized racism of African American children. Her doll studies highlighted the harm done to children in segregated schools and were instrumental in the 1954 *Brown v. Board of Education* court case. In 1946, Clark co-founded the Northside Center for Child Development. This center was the first to offer therapy to children in Harlem and focused on children of color and low socioeconomic status. The therapists at the center utilized multicultural modalities to work with children in a holistic manner.

Lillian Comas-Diaz

Lillian Comas-Diaz was born in Chicago and raised in Puerto Rico. After earning her graduate degree in clinical psychology, she began to address the need for psychology to consider marginalized and underserved populations. She helped found the American Psychological Association's Society for the Psychological Study of Culture, Ethnicity, and Race. Comas-Diaz also developed a feminist liberation model that can be used in psychological work.

Jennifer Eberhardt

Jennifer Eberhardt (1965–present) was born in Cleveland, Ohio. She earned her doctorate in psychology from Harvard University. Her work includes a focus on "investigating the subtle, complex, largely unconscious yet deeply ingrained ways that individuals racially code and categorize people, with a particular focus on associations between race and crime" (MacArthur Foundation, 2014). Her work on racial bias and inequality has been recognized with various awards.

Olivia Espín

Olivia Espín (1938–present) was born in Cuba and earned her doctorate from the University of Florida in 1974. Her research focuses on race and sexuality particularly in immigrant and Latina women.

Evelyn Hooker

Evelyn Hooker (1907–1996) was born in North Platte, Nebraska. Hooker was instrumental in challenging the stigmatization of homosexuality as a mental disorder. She earned her doctorate in psychology from Johns Hopkins University in 1932. Her research centered on gay men and showed that they did not possess abnormal pathology and, therefore, were not mentally ill. She later became the chair of National Institute of Mental Health Task Force on Homosexuality and issued reports recommending the repeal of "sodomy laws, portrayed employment discrimination as a problem, and called for better public education" (Ware, 2005, p. 309). She played a fundamental role in the American Psychological Association's decision to remove homosexuality from the list of mental disorders in 1973 (Ware, 2005).

Margaret Jeannette Naumburg

Margaret Jeannette Naumburg (1890–1983) was born in New York City. Naumburg is credited by many with creating art therapy. She was the first psychologist to train students in art therapy in the United States. She created analytically oriented art therapy, which held that the subconscious could communicate through artistic expression.

Mary Cover Jones

Mary Cover Jones (1897–1987) was born in Johnstown, Pennsylvania, to a homemaker mother and businessman father. Her father did not attend university and encouraged Jones to attend Vassar College, where she majored in psychology. After graduating from Vassar, Jones attended a lecture by John B. Watson, the father of behaviorism psychology. This lecture set in motion Jones's behavioral work centered on reducing and eliminating fears, also known as desensitization. Jones published a study of "Little Peter." Her findings contradicted John B. Watson's classical conditioning findings indicating that "Little Albert" could be conditioned to display a fear response. Little Peter had a fear reduced by use of direct conditioning.

Jill Holly Freedman

Jill Holly Freedman (1951–present) works as a narrative therapist, supervisor, consultant, and trainer. She has been involved in almost all aspects of narrative therapy for more than three decades. Freedman received her master's degree in social work from Washington University in St. Louis in 1975; she then intensively studied family therapy with Michael White and David Epston. She is codirector of the Evanston Family Therapy Center, an independent postgraduate training center dedicated to teaching narrative therapy. She is a founding member of the Chicago Center for Family Health and is on the international faculty of the Dulwich Centre in Adelaide, Australia. Along with her partner, Gene Combs, she has coauthored three books and more than thirty book chapters and articles about narrative therapy. She is internationally recognized for her contributions to narrative therapy, having presented her work on every continent but Antarctica.

Inez Beverly Prosser

Inez Beverly Prosser (1895–1934) was born in Yoakum, Texas, and was the first African American woman to earn a doctorate in psychology in the United States. Her work focused on the impact of segregated schools on African American children. She argued that African American children's psyches were impacted by racial injustices and isolation.

Beverly Daniel Tatum

Beverly Daniel Tatum (1954–present) was born in Tallahassee, Florida. Tatum earned her doctorate in clinical psychology from the University of Michigan in 1984. Her work included racial identity development and the topic of race in education. She utilized racial identity models when making sense of people's reactions to her work as a diversity trainer and educator.

Reiko True

Reiko True (1933–present) was born in Japan and moved to the United States in 1958. She is best known as an advocate for mental health services for Asian Americans and other marginalized populations. She was a founding member of the Asian American Psychological Association.

Ena Vazquez-Nuttall

Ena Vazquez-Nuttall was born in Puerto Rico and earned her doctorate in education with a focus on counseling and school psychology from Boston University. She is best known for studying and teaching cultural diversity before it was considered significant in the fields of counseling and psychology.

THEMES

The women highlighted in this book are but a few of the theorists that we have been able to uncover in our quest to amplify women's voices. There are common threads found in and among the women theorists. One of the themes we found as characteristic of these women theorists is that of a resistance to or in some cases a rejection of family expectations and family legacy. We also noticed the use of personal experiences as a catalyst for their theoretical development. It is interesting to note that these first two themes, rejection of family legacy and personal experiences dovetail nicely with the political argument used as a rallying slogan of the second-wave feminism from the late 1960s that the personal is political. These women theorists were challenging the social structures, values, and norms; the Eurocentric status quo created by White men that have maintained power of the western world for centuries. We have come full circle to the reason we wrote this book, that women's contributions were silenced by the Eurocentric values and beliefs that are pervasive throughout theory of human psychology and counseling.

Other themes we noticed with the women theorists portrayed in this book is the expansion of initial theories to include more groups. Not only in therapeutic practice, but also in the academy as a whole. Many women theorists established committees and organizations devoted to understanding marginalized groups' experiences. The result is a more wholistic multifaceted approach to human psychological concepts and behaviors. Spirituality in some form was a theme with many women, such as the impact of religious persecution and connecting to people on a spiritual level. The theme of negotiation of professional identity within the context of marriage was prevalent. Each woman distinguished themselves from their husbands in some way, whether within their marriage, during their husband's lives or after the marriage ended either through divorce or death.

Understanding these themes is important for continuing to recover women's voices. There are those who are not in this edition of the book, but we are continuing to investigate, recover, and amplify forgotten women's voices. These themes are important for the present-day women who are experiencing the silencing of their voice and ideas. We want to ensure that the women who are active now are not forgotten. We continue to promote and support women who are at the forefront of theory development, creating new ways of understanding our individual selves and us as a collective culture of a diversity of voices, all of whom are heard.

REFERENCES

American Psychological Association (2012). Ena Vazquez-Nuttall: Featured psychologist. https://www.apa.org/pi/oema/resources/ethnicity-health/psychologists/vazquez-nuttall

American Psychological Association (2012). Reiko True, PhD: Featured psychologist. https://www.apa.org/pi/oema/resources/ethnicity-health/psychologists/true

American Psychological Association. (2012). Carolyn Lewis Attneave, PhD. https://www.apa.org/pi/oema/resources/ethnicity-health/psychologists/carolyn-lewis-attneave

Bernal, M. (2001). Award for distinguished contributions to the public interest. *American Psychologist*, 56(11), 922–924. doi:10.1037/0003-066X.56.11.922b

George, M. (2019). Carolyn Attneave. *Feminist Voices*. http://www.feministvoices.com/carolyn-attneave/

Harutyunyan, A., & Horschelmann, K. (2009). *Public Spheres After Socialism*. Intellect Books.

Jones, B. D. (2017). Askwith Essentials: Who is Beverly Daniel Tatum? *Harvard Graduate School of Education*. https://www.gse.harvard.edu/news/17/03/askwith-essentials-who-beverly-daniel-tatum

Kawahara, D. M. (2017). The amazing life and times of Oliva Espín. *Women & Therapy*, *40*(34), 323–333. doi:10.1080/02703149.2017.1241571

Lebow, J., Chambers, A., & Breunlin, D. C. (eds.). (2019). *Encyclopedia of Couple and Family Therapy*. Springer International Publishing.

Lewis, R. (2011). Profile: Olivia Espín. *Feminist Voices*. http://www.feministvoices.com/olivaespin/

Logan, D. (1980). Mary Cover Jones: Feminine as asset. *Psychology of Women Quarterly*, *5*(1), 103–115. doi:10.1111/j.1471-6402.1980.tb01037.x

Ludy Jr., B. T. (2008). America's first black female psychologist. *American Psychological Association*. https://www.apa.org/monitor/2008/11/prosser

Mussen, P., & Eichorn, D. (1988). Mary Cover Jones (1896–1987). *American Psychologist*, *43*(10), 818. doi:10.1037/h0091933

Rutherford, A. (2010). Profile: Mary Cover Jones. *Psychology's Feminist Voices*. http://www.feministvoices.com/mary-cover-jones/

Stanford University (n.d.). About Jennifer Lynn Eberhardt. *Department of Psychology*. https://web.stanford.edu/~eberhard/about-jennifer-eberhardt.html

Vasquez, M. T., & Lopez, S. (2002). Martha E. Bernal (1931–2001). *American Psychologist*, *57*(5), 362–363. doi:10.1037/0003-066X.57.5.362

Ware, S. (2005). *Notable American Women: A Biographical Dictionary Completing the Twentieth Century* (Vol. 5). Belknap Press of Harvard University Press.

Glossary

Theodora Mead Abel
Mary Ainsworth
Louise Bates Ames
Carolyn Attneave
Virginia Axline
Insoo Kim Berg
Martha Bernal
Mamie Phipps Clark
Lillian Comas-Diaz
Jennifer Eberhardt
Olivia Espín
Jill Holly Freedman
Anna Freud
Carol Gilligan
Evelyn Hooker
Karen Horney
Mary Cover Jones
Melanie Klein
Kimberlé Crenshaw
Margaret Mahler
Jean Baker Miller
Margaret Jeannette Naumburg
Laura Perls
Inez Beverly Prosser
Natalie Rogers

Virginia Satir
Beverly Daniel Tatum
Reiko True
Ena Vazquez-Nuttall
Cheryl White

Index

About the Authors

Lynn Bohecker, Ph.D., LMFT is an associate professor in the Department of Counseling and Family Studies at Liberty University. She graduated from Idaho State University with a doctorate in Counselor Education and Counseling. Her research interests include feminist pedagogy, group work, spirituality integration into counseling and advocacy. Dr. Bohecker is the director at The Counseling Center at Tree City Church. She has published in peer-reviewed journals such as Feminist Teacher, The Qualitative Report, Journal of LGBT Issues in Counseling, Counselor Education & Supervision, Journal for Specialists in Group Work, and Journal for Counseling & Development. Dr. Bohecker has also written several book chapters in counseling related publications.

Kirsten LaMantia, PhD, LPC, NCC, is an associate professor in the Department of Psychology and Counseling at Southeast Missouri State University. Dr. LaMantia is a licensed professional counselor in the state of Missouri. Dr. LaMantia serves as the Mental Health Program Coordinator and Counseling Clinic Director. Dr. LaMantia's research interests are in multicultural competence in counseling settings. These topics include cross-cultural counseling, values bracketing, and counseling marginalized populations. In addition, Dr. LaMantia explores issues concerning local, regional, and national advocacy for marginalized populations. Additionally, Dr. LaMantia conducts research on feminist pedagogy within the counseling field, has many international and national presentations and scholarly publications.

Holly Wagner, PhD, LPC, NCC, is an associate professor in the Department of Psychology and Counseling. Dr. Wagner's specialty area is School Counseling, with areas of concentration including Career Development,

Human Growth & Development, Helping Relationships, and Professional Orientation & Ethics. She is a nationally certified counselor and a licensed professional counselor in Missouri. Dr. Wagner serves as the Play Therapy Education Coordinator for the Play Therapy Sequence in the Department of Psychology and Counseling. Dr. Wagner has previous work experience as a Professional School Counselor in a K-8 school setting, the program leader for the school counseling track at Montana State University, and an assistant professor at the University of Missouri-Saint Louis. Dr. Wagner's research interests include school counseling, play therapy, trauma-informed counseling, counselor development, feminist pedagogy, cultural competence, LGBTQQIA competence and advocacy, and social justice issues in counselor education. She is publishing in journals such as Counselor Education & Supervision, Journal of LGBT Issues in Counseling, and the Journal of School Counseling. She looks forward to continued research and scholarship that impact clinical, programmatic, pedagogical, and supervisory domains within the fields of counseling, school counseling, and counselor education.

About the Contributors

TeShaunda Hannor-Walker, PhD, LPC, NCC, CPCS is an assistant graduate professor at Liberty University, a Licensed Clinical Therapist, and author of *How to Raise a Successful Child with ADD.* She served fifteen years in the public schools and was named, The American School Counselor Association's "Top Ten School Counselors in America." She is also a National Certified Counselor (NCC) and Licensed Professional Counselor (LPC). Dr. Hannor-Walker has presented at local, state, and national conferences for over a decade on various counseling topics.

Carol Robinson is a psychotherapist specializing in individual, couples and family therapy maintaining a private practice in Saint Louis, Missouri. With over twenty years of experience working with individual and group clients to clarify current challenges and future goals, Carol currently works with a broad spectrum of clients. In addition to being a prominent relationship therapist, she presents at National conferences and to general audiences speaking on the topics of Stress Management, Mental Health for Busy Professionals, Cultural Diversity in Counseling, Spirituality and Lesbian, Gay, Bisexual and Transgender counseling. Carol has received specialized training as a Psychodynamic Psychotherapist in addition to training in a broad range of therapies.

www.ingramcontent.com/pod-product-compliance
Ingram Content Group UK Ltd.
Pitfield, Milton Keynes, MK11 3LW, UK
UKHW041844031026
15587UKWH00003B/995

9 781793 608475